Primary Total Ankle Replacement

Editor

THOMAS S. ROUKIS

CLINICS IN PODIATRIC MEDICINE AND SURGERY

www.podiatric.theclinics.com

Consulting Editor
THOMAS ZGONIS

January 2013 • Volume 30 • Number 1

ELSEVIER

1600 John F. Kennedy Boulevard • Suite 1800 • Philadelphia, Pennsylvania 19103-2899

http://www.theclinics.com

CLINICS IN PODIATRIC MEDICINE AND SURGERY Volume 30, Number 1
January 2013 ISSN 0891-8422, ISBN-13: 978-1-4557-7142-4

Editor: Patrick Manley

Clinics in Podiatric Medicine and Surgery (ISSN 0891-8422) is published quarterly by Elsevier Inc., 360 Park Avenue South, New York, NY 10010-1710. Months of issue are January, April, July, and October. Business and Editorial Offices: 1600 John F. Kennedy Blvd., Ste. 1800, Philadelphia, PA 19103-2899. Customer Service Office: 3251 Riverport Lane, Maryland Heights, MO 63043. Periodicals postage paid at New York, NY and additional mailing offices. Subscription prices are $292.00 per year for US individuals, $410.00 per year for US institutions, $148.00 per year for US students and residents, $350.00 per year for Canadian individuals, $508.00 for Canadian institutions, $415.00 for international individuals, $508.00 per year for international institutions and $208.00 per year for Canadian and foreign students/residents. To receive student/resident rate, orders must be accompanied by name of affiliated institution, date of term, and the *signature* of program/residency coordinator on institution letterhead. Orders will be billed at individual rate until proof of status is received. Foreign air speed delivery is included in all *Clinics* subscription prices. All prices are subject to change without notice. POSTMASTER: Send address changes to *Clinics in Podiatric Medicine and Surgery*, Elsevier Health Sciences Division, Subscription Customer Service, 3251 Riverport Lane, Maryland Heights, MO 63043. **Customer Service: 1-800-654-2452 (US). From outside of the US, call 314-447-8871. Fax: 314-447-8029. E-mail: JournalsCustomerService-usa@elsevier.com (for print support); JournalsOnlineSupport-usa@elsevier.com (for online support).**

Reprints. For copies of 100 or more of articles in this publication, please contact the Commercial Reprints Department, Elsevier Inc., 360 Park Avenue South, New York, NY 10010-1710. Tel.: 212-633-3812; Fax: 212-462-1935; E-mail: reprints@elsevier.com.

Clinics in Podiatric Medicine and Surgery is covered in *MEDLINE/PubMed (Index Medicus)* and *EMBASE/Excerpta Medica.*

Printed and bound by CPI Group (UK) Ltd, Croydon, CR0 4YY

Transferred to digital print 2012

CLINICS IN PODIATRIC MEDICINE AND SURGERY

Contributors

CONSULTING EDITOR

THOMAS ZGONIS, DPM, FACFAS
Associate Professor, Fellowship Director in Reconstructive Foot and Ankle Surgery and Chief, Division of Podiatric Medicine and Surgery, Department of Orthopaedic Surgery, University of Texas Health Science Center at San Antonio, San Antonio, Texas

GUEST EDITOR

THOMAS S. ROUKIS, DPM, PhD, FACFAS
Attending Staff, Department of Orthopaedics, Podiatry, and Sports Medicine, Gundersen Lutheran Healthcare System, La Crosse, Wisconsin

AUTHORS

BRADLEY P. ABICHT, DPM, AACFAS
Attending Staff, Department of Orthopaedics, Podiatry, and Sports Medicine, Gundersen Lutheran Healthcare System, La Crosse, Wisconsin

GREGORY C. BERLET, MD
Orthopedic Foot and Ankle Center, Westerville, Ohio

CHRISTOPHER BIBBO, DO, DPM, FACS, FAAOS, FACFAS
Chief, Foot & Ankle Section, Department of Orthopaedics, Marshfield Clinic, Marshfield, Wisconsin

SARA L. BORKOSKY, DPM
Podiatric Medicine and Surgery Resident, PGY-III, Gundersen Lutheran Medical Foundation, La Crosse, Wisconsin

WOO JIN CHOI, MD
Department of Orthopaedic Surgery, Yonsei University College of Medicine, Seoul, South Korea

JAMES K. DEORIO, MD
Associate Professor, Department of Orthopedics, Duke University, Durham, North Carolina

J. GEORGE DEVRIES, DPM, AACFAS
Associate of the American College of Foot and Ankle Surgeons, Excel Orthopedics, Beaver Dam, Wisconsin

NIKOLAOS GOUGOULIAS, MD, PhD
Consultant Orthopaedic Foot & Ankle Surgeon, Department of Trauma and Orthopaedics, Frimley Park Hospital, Camberley, Surrey, United Kingdom

CHRISTOPHER F. HYER, DPM, MS, FACFAS
Orthopedic Foot and Ankle Center, Westerville, Ohio

JIN WOO LEE, MD, PhD
Department of Orthopaedic Surgery, Yonsei University College of Medicine, Seoul, South Korea

THOMAS H. LEE, MD
Orthopedic Foot and Ankle Center, Westerville, Ohio

NICOLA MAFFULLI, MD, MS, PhD, FRCP, FRCS(Orth), FFSEM
Centre Lead and Professor of Sports and Exercise Medicine, Consultant Trauma and Orthopaedic Surgeon, Barts and The London School of Medicine and Dentistry, William Harvey Research Institute, Mile End Hospital, Queen Mary University of London, London, United Kingdom

MICHAEL MANKOVECKY, DPM
Podiatric Medicine and Surgery Resident, PGY-II, Gundersen Lutheran Medical Foundation, La Crosse, Wisconsin

MARK PRISSEL, DPM
Podiatric Medicine and Surgery Resident, PGY-II, Gundersen Lutheran Medical Foundation, La Crosse, Wisconsin

THOMAS S. ROUKIS, DPM, PhD, FACFAS
Attending Staff, Department of Orthopaedics, Podiatry, and Sports Medicine, Gundersen Lutheran Healthcare System, La Crosse, Wisconsin

SHANNON M. RUSH, DPM, FACFAS
Director, Silicon Valley Foot and Ankle Fellowship, Department of Podiatric Surgery, Palo Alto Medical Foundation; Vice Chief, Department of Podiatric Surgery, El Camino Hospital, Mountain View, California

BRYAN A. SAGRAY, DPM
Instructor/Clinical and Fellow in Reconstructive Foot and Ankle Surgery, Division of Podiatric Medicine and Surgery, Department of Orthopaedic Surgery, University of Texas Health Science Center at San Antonio, San Antonio, Texas

RYAN T. SCOTT, DPM, AACFAS
Associate of the American College of Foot and Ankle Surgeons, Orthopedic Foot and Ankle Center, Westerville, Ohio

JOHN J. STAPLETON, DPM, FACFAS
Associate, Foot and Ankle Surgery, VSAS Orthopaedics and Chief of Podiatric Surgery, Lehigh Valley Hospital, Cedar Crest Campus, Allentown, Pennsylvania; Clinical Assistant Professor of Surgery, Penn State College of Medicine, Hershey, Pennsylvania

NICHOLAS TODD, DPM, AACFAS
Department of Podiatric Surgery, Palo Alto Medical Foundation, Mountain View, California

HANG SEOB YOON, MD
Department of Orthopaedic Surgery, Yonsei University College of Medicine, Seoul, South Korea

THOMAS ZGONIS, DPM, FACFAS
Associate Professor, Fellowship Director in Reconstructive Foot and Ankle Surgery and Chief, Division of Podiatric Medicine and Surgery, Department of Orthopaedic Surgery, University of Texas Health Science Center at San Antonio, San Antonio, Texas

Contents

> Attempts at ankle replacement have existed for at least 50 years. Time has essentially eliminated constrained, cemented, first-generation ankle replacements. Although some two-component, more anatomic, designs are still used with varying success, three-component "mobile bearing" ankle prostheses are winning the race of evolution. Not only have implants change over the years, but also the patients and surgeons. Surgeons specialize, improving their surgical outcomes and expanding the indications for total ankle replacement in technically demanding complex ankles. High-demand, younger patients, but also obese ones, are potential candidates for a total ankle replacement. This article provides a review of the history of total ankle replacement.

> Although there exist general guidelines regarding which patients are "suitable" candidates for total ankle replacement, these guidelines tend to be very conservative, much like those of knee and hip replacement from decades ago. There are also no direct comparison studies of one total ankle replacement design with another. Because of the paucity of data, surgeons are left to surmise the opinion based on limited studies, as well as industry-sponsored data and advertising material. This article examines several key, controversial issues that apply to total ankle replacement. Recommendations and points for thought are provided.

> The ultimate goal of primary total ankle replacement is to provide a well-balanced soft-tissue envelope around a well-aligned, well-fixated implant. Some surgeons have emphasized that good outcomes in total ankle replacement are more dependent on ligament balancing, along with the procedure itself, than the extent of preoperative coronal deformity in the ankle. Thus, it is imperative that the surgeon be familiar with additional procedures to address the varus, valgus, and other associated deformities commonly encountered in primary total ankle replacement.

Current Concepts and Techniques in Foot and Ankle Surgery

Thomas S. Roukis

This article presents a procedure whereby a second-phase design DePuy Alvine Total Ankle Prosthesis underwent revision to an Agility LP custom-designed stemmed tibial and talar component total ankle replacement system. The rationale for this procedure, the process of developing the custom components, the operative sequence of events, and recovery course are presented in detail. Causes for concern regarding subsequent revision, should this be required, are raised.

Bryan A. Sagray, John J. Stapleton, and Thomas Zgonis

Calcaneal fractures among the diabetic population are severe and complex injuries that warrant careful evaluation in an effort to carry out adequate conservative or surgical management. The complication rates associated with diabetic fracture management are increased and may include poor wound healing, deep infection, malunion, and Charcot neuroarthropathy, each of which can pose a risk for limb loss. The significant surgery-associated morbidity accompanying diabetic calcaneal fractures has led to improved methods of calcaneal fracture management. This article reviews the overall management of diabetic calcaneal fractures, complications, and outcomes.

CLINICS IN PODIATRIC MEDICINE AND SURGERY

FORTHCOMING ISSUES

April 2013
Revision Total Ankle Replacement
Thomas S. Roukis, DPM, *Guest Editor*

July 2013
Advances in Forefoot Surgery
Charles Zelen, DPM, *Guest Editor*

August 2013
Pediatric Foot Deformities
Patrick DeHeer, DPM, *Guest Editor*

RECENT ISSUES

October 2012
Ankle Arthritis
Jess Burks, DPM, *Guest Editor*

July 2012
**Contemporary Controversies in
Foot & Ankle Surgery**
Neal M. Blitz, DPM, *Guest Editor*

April 2012
Foot and Ankle Trauma
Denise Mandi, DPM, *Guest Editor*

Foreword
Primary Total Ankle Replacement

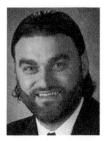

Thomas Zgonis, DPM, FACFAS
Consulting Editor

This edition of *Clinics in Podiatric Medicine and Surgery* is focused on the indications and surgical options for primary total ankle replacement available in the United States. Total ankle replacement is becoming more popular in the recent years, addressing primary degenerative joint and posttraumatic ankle deformities. A detailed review of each available ankle replacement implant with its indications and management of concomitant foot and ankle deformities is addressed by the invited authors.

The guest editor, Dr Roukis, has done an outstanding job of selecting national and international experts in the surgical field of total ankle replacement. His scientific contributions and expertise in the realm of foot and ankle surgery are well recognized by his peers. Dr Roukis will also guest edit the April 2013 edition of *Clinics in Podiatric Medicine and Surgery* devoted to Revision Total Ankle Replacement. I hope that you will find both editions helpful when you encounter patients undergoing primary and revision total ankle replacement.

Thomas Zgonis, DPM, FACFAS
Division of Podiatric Medicine and Surgery
Department of Orthopaedic Surgery
University of Texas Health Science Center San Antonio
7703 Floyd Curl Drive-MSC 7776
San Antonio, TX 78229, USA

E-mail address:
zgonis@uthscsa.edu

Clin Podiatr Med Surg 30 (2013) xi
http://dx.doi.org/10.1016/j.cpm.2012.09.004 **podiatric.theclinics.com**

Preface

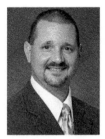

Thomas S. Roukis, DPM, PhD, FACFAS
Guest Editor

It is with great pleasure that I serve as guest editor for this issue of *Clinics in Podiatric Medicine and Surgery* devoted to "Primary Total Ankle Replacement." The intent of this issue is to provide up-to-date information available for contemporary total ankle replacement devices with an emphasis on those available in the United States. Surprisingly few textbooks or clinics issues devoted to this topic exist and many of those that do are outdated or involve total ankle replacement systems no longer available for use or ones that are not available for use in the United States. The international authors selected are respected authorities on the topics they have been assigned and have been gracious enough to take substantial time from their practices and families to accommodate my tight and in many ways unrealistic goals for this issue.

At the time of this publication, 4 total ankle replacements systems are readily available for use in the United States: Agility and Agility LP (DePuy Orthopaedics, Warsaw, IN); INBONE, INBONE II, and Prophecy (Wright Medical Technology, Arlington, TN); Salto Talaris (Tornier, Inc, Bloomington, MN); and STAR (Small Bone Innovations, Inc, Morrisville, PA). Following a detailed review of the history of total ankle replacement, we discuss a number of controversies germane to our current understanding of total ankle replacement. A detailed review of techniques useful for predictably managing varus and valgus deformities present preoperatively follows. Much has been written about the Agility and STAR total ankle replacement systems for primary implantation and accordingly we instead focus on the INBONE prostheses and Salto Talaris total ankle replacement systems. This is a prelude to the April 2013 issue devoted entirely to "Revision Total Ankle Replacement."

Clin Podiatr Med Surg 30 (2013) xiii–xiv
http://dx.doi.org/10.1016/j.cpm.2012.09.003
0891-8422/13/$ – see front matter © 2013 Elsevier Inc. All rights reserved.

podiatric.theclinics.com

It is hoped that the readers of this issue of *Clinics of Podiatric Medicine and Surgery* will enjoy these articles and benefit from the surgical experience of the authors selected as much as I have.

Thomas S. Roukis, DPM, PhD, FACFAS
Department of Orthopaedics, Podiatry, and Sports Medicine
Gundersen Lutheran Healthcare System
La Crosse, WI, USA

E-mail address:
tsroukis@gundluth.org

History of Total Ankle Replacement

Nikolaos Gougoulias, MD, PhD[a],
Nicola Maffulli, MD, MS, PhD, FRCP, FRCS(Orth), FFSEM[b,*]

KEYWORDS

• Arthroplasty • Joint pain • Joint replacement • Tibio-talar joint

KEY POINTS

• Ankle arthroplasty remains a challenging procedure, given the unique kinematic and anatomic characteristics of the hindfoot.
• Nonconstrained, three-component, mobile-bearing implants reduce friction and polyethylene wear.
• Cementless with bone ongrowth is superior to polymethyl methacrylate cement fixation.
• Technological advances may enhance bone ingrowth onto the implant surfaces.
• Specialized centers and individual surgeons performing a high-volume of total ankle replacements provide superior outcomes.
• The survivorship of total ankle replacements is inferior to that of knee and hip replacements.
• Systematic reviews and long-term cohort studies may provide useful conclusions, highlighting failures of certain implants and techniques.

INTRODUCTION

The first reported attempt to avoid fusion of an arthritic ankle was in 1913 when Eloesser[1] performed ankle cartilage allograft transplantation. A "hemi-arthroplasty" of the ankle joint, using a custom vitallium talar dome resurfacing implant, was performed in a 31-year-old man in 1962. The patient was a heavy laborer, suffering from posttraumatic arthritis after a Weber-C ankle fracture, who did not respond to nonoperative management. His surgeon, Carrol Larson, applied the concept of "cup arthroplasty" of the hip popularized at the time by his mentor, Smith-Petersen, in the ankle. A talar dome replacing prosthesis was implanted through a lateral

[a] Department of Trauma and Orthopaedics, Frimley Park Hospital, Portsmouth Road, Camberley, Surrey, GU16 7UJ, UK; [b] Queen Mary University of London, Barts and The London School of Medicine and Dentistry, William Harvey Research Institute, Centre for Sports and Exercise Medicine, Mile End Hospital, 275 Bancroft Road, London E1 4DG, UK
* Corresponding author.
E-mail address: n.maffulli@qmul.ac.uk

Clin Podiatr Med Surg 30 (2013) 1–20
http://dx.doi.org/10.1016/j.cpm.2012.08.005   **podiatric.theclinics.com**
0891-8422/13/$ – see front matter © 2013 Elsevier Inc. All rights reserved.

approach. The patient was able to bear full weight 3-months postoperatively and continued to work in a factory as a heavy laborer for many years. Against all odds, the "primitive" implant survived, and 40 years later, at the age of 71 years, the patient presented for follow-up with minimal hindfoot malalignment and no symptoms.[2]

The first "total" ankle replacement was performed by Lord and Marrotte in 1970.[3] Their prosthesis could be described as a "reverse hip," with a long stem metallic component implanted into the tibia, articulating with a cemented acetabular cup in the calcaneus, after the talus had been completely removed.[3] After 25 ankle replacements with the "reverse hip prosthesis," the implant was abandoned because of unsatisfactory results.[3]

Learning from failure, surgeons continued to modify implant designs, moving from constrained to less constrained, and from two- to three-component mobile-bearing designs (**Figs. 1** and **2**).[4] Outcomes seem to gradually improve, with survivorship rates of approximately 80% at 10 years.[5]

The stimulus for total ankle replacement in the last 42 years derived from partial dissatisfaction with ankle arthrodesis[4,6–9] and the success of total hip and knee arthroplasties.[10,11] The rationale was to reduce friction, which produces polyethylene wear leading to loosening, at the same time taking into consideration the unique biomechanical characteristics and kinematics of the joints of the hindfoot.[12–15] Over the years, the use of polymethyl methacrylate cement for implant fixation was abandoned, whereas advancements in technology led to improved metallic implant surfaces that could induce bone ongrowth and reduce aseptic loosening (**Fig. 3**). Current total ankle

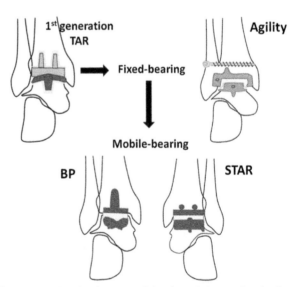

Fig. 1. Most first-generation implants used in the 1970s consisted of an all ultrahigh-molecular-weight polyethylene (UHMWPE) tibial component and were fixed with cement. The next generation included a UHMWPE component fixed onto the tibial tray. Designs moved from constrained to semiconstrained, the Agility prosthesis being an example. The Buechel-Pappas (BP) and the Scandinavian Total Ankle Replacement (STAR) contain a mobile-bearing UHMWPE insert (three-component implants), allowing sliding motion on either side of the UHMWPE toward the tibial and the talar components, respectively. Polymethyl methacrylate cement fixation was gradually abandoned. The BP uses a tibial stem for stabilization, whereas the STAR is fixed through hollow bars. Newer three-component designs have adapted features from the BP and the STAR prostheses.

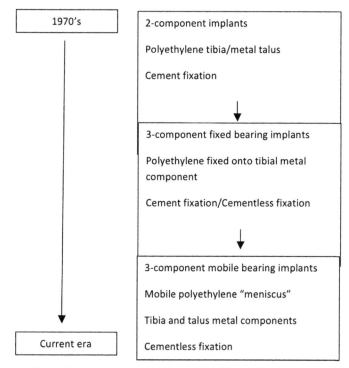

1970's	2-component implants
	Polyethylene tibia/metal talus
	Cement fixation

3-component fixed bearing implants

Polyethylene fixed onto tibial metal component

Cement fixation/Cementless fixation

3-component mobile bearing implants

Mobile polyethylene "meniscus"

Tibia and talus metal components

| Current era | Cementless fixation |

Fig. 2. Total ankle replacement. Evolution from the 1970s to the current era.

replacement systems include various materials and shapes of fixation elements. Pegs, long or short stems, and cylindrical or rectangular bars have been used. Replacement of medial and lateral gutters varies among different designs.[4] Cobalt-chromium alloy is the current material of choice for total ankle prostheses. All popular total ankle replacements are composed of titanium or cobalt chromium, except for the Takakura Nara Kyocera (TNK; Kyocera, Kyoto, Japan). This is a ceramic prosthesis used predominantly in Japan.[16] A recent development is the combination of cobalt-chromium with a ceramic titanium nitride coating, the so called "BONIT coating" (porous coating with titanium plasma sprayed surface and an additional layer of calcium phosphate) of metallic components to enhance osteointegration.[4] Advances in instrumentation and prosthesis design try to minimize bone resection for implantation of the prosthesis.[4,17,18]

However, despite continuous modifications and improvements, the survivorship rate of ankle replacements, according to data from national joint registers[19–28] and clinical studies,[5] is still lagging behind that of hip and knee replacements, with failure rates for replaced ankles approximately double compared with hips and knees.[11,12] The reason may be the complexity of structure and function of the ankle joint.[12–15]

This article describes key features of historical implants no longer in use, and how prosthesis designs evolved over the years. It also examines how clinical outcomes have changed, and how and why indications for total ankle replacement have expanded.

HISTORICAL TOTAL ANKLE REPLACEMENT DESIGNS

The first ankle implant replacements were performed in the 1970s. Prostheses of this era were mostly constrained, consisting of two-components (the tibia and the talar

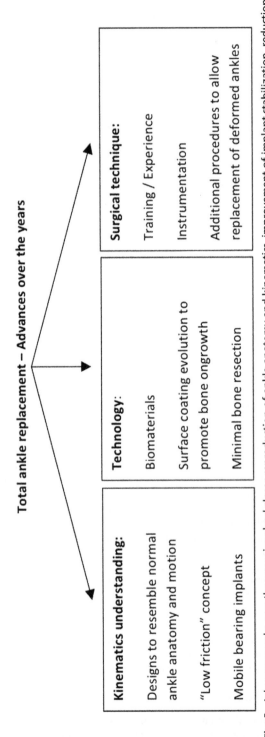

Fig. 3. Advances made over the years involved closer reproduction of ankle anatomy and kinematics, improvement of implant stabilization, reduction of UHMWPE wear, surgical technique, and expansion of indications.

components, without "meniscal" bearing), requiring polymethyl methacrylate cement fixation (see **Fig. 1**). High rates of implant aseptic loosening, pain, and revision to fusion were reported.[4] They were abandoned as surgeons started to recognize their limitations and moved on to design total ankle replacements that could reproduce the "natural" ankle kinematics.

Lord and Marrotte implanted the first total ankle arthroplasty, a simple "hinged" design, in 1970.[3] A long stem tibial component (similar to a femoral prosthesis) articulated with a polyethylene talar body replacing component, fixed into the calcaneus. Only 7 out of 25 arthroplasties gave satisfactory results, 12 implants had failed at 10 years, and the use of the prosthesis was abandoned. It was realized at the time that an element of rotation is essential for natural hindfoot movement.

Almost in parallel, surgeons in Sweden implanted the St. George prosthesis (semi-constrained, implanted through a lateral approach), in 1973. Only eight ankle replacements were performed before the implant was abandoned, because of the high rate of early complications.[29,30]

Another two-component constrained design, the Imperial College of London Hospital prosthesis, was used from 1972 to 1981.[31,32] It required polymethyl methacrylate cemented fixation, and contained a polyethylene tibial implant. The tibial component had raised medial and lateral walls to prevent subluxation of the talar component.[31] Half of the implants were converted to fusion at 5.5 years, and only 11 out of 62 ankles yielded satisfactory results. Pain, wound healing problems, talar collapse, and loosening of the components were common, bringing Bolton-Maggs and colleagues[32] to state that "…it is a matter of time before all prosthesis fail and require arthrodesis."

The Irvine nonconstrained implant (Howmedica, Rutherford, NJ) was used in California in the 1970s.[33] It was probably the first design that attempted to reproduce the shape of the talus, based on anatomic studies. They aimed to achieve motion in the sagittal and coronal planes, at the same time allowing axial rotation. It was realized later, however, that rotation increased stresses on the ligaments.[34] The designers reported two early failures after 28 arthroplasties were performed. Malalignment was common, and no further report regarding the Irvine implant ever followed.

Another early era constrained implant, the CONAXIAL Beck-Steffe, showed 60% loosening at 5 years and up to 90% at 10 years[35] and was abandoned. A similarly highly congruent two-component implant from the 1970s is the Mayo Total Ankle Replacement, designed by Stauffer and Segal.[36] It contained a polyethylene tibia component and required polymethyl methacrylate cement fixation. Kitaoka and colleagues[37,38] reported on the long-term outcome of the prosthesis, reviewing 204 ankle arthroplasties performed in 179 patients at the Mayo Clinic from 1974 to 1988. Good results were obtained in 19% of the patients. Implant removal was required in 36%, 94 reoperations were needed, and aseptic loosening of the talar component was common. The cumulative survival rates of 79%, 65%, and 61%, at 5, 10, and 15 years, respectively, highlighted the problems related to the use of constrained implants.[37,38]

The Newton Ankle Implant (Howmedica, Rutherford, NJ) was an incongruous cemented two-component prosthesis used in the late 1970s. The polyethylene tibial component was a portion of a cylinder, whereas the spherical talar component had a slightly smaller radius. This resulted in increased polyethylene wear and a 75% rate of aseptic loosening. At 3 years, only 38% of 34 prostheses remained in situ.[39]

The Richard Smith ankle arthroplasty (Dow Corning, Arlington, TN) had incongruent surfaces. Clinical results showed failure rates of 29% at 7 years.[40]

The use of the Bath-Wessex total ankle replacement, a two-component (polyethylene tibia) nonconstrained polymethyl methacrylate cemented design, was documented in 72 ankles from 1984 to 1996.[41] Survival rates sharply decreased from 83% at 5 years to 66% at 10 years. Radiographic loosening was very common (47% in the tibia and 82% in the talus at 10 years).[41]

The Thompson-Richard prosthesis, introduced in 1976, was a cemented, two-component, semiconstrained prosthesis only allowing plantarflexion and dorsiflexion. The concave polyethylene tibial component had a lip on each side restricting side-to-side movement of the talus. Therefore, shear forces were transmitted to the bone-cement interface. This resulted in 52% radiolucency and 69% satisfaction rate at 5 years, although only 2 out of 30 implants were removed.[42] High survival (87%) and high radiolucency rates (53%) were reported by other authors at 12-years follow-up.[43] Pain was very common, with low functional scoring, according to another study.[44] The Norwegian Joint Registry revealed a 19% revision rate at 7.7 years in 32 ankles from 1994 to 1997.[21] The use of this prosthesis has not been documented after 1997.

The New Jersey ankle replacement was developed by Frederick Buechel, an ortho-pedic surgeon, and Michael Pappas, a bioengineer, and was the predecessor of modern ankle arthroplasty implants. It was first implanted in 1974, and had a similar fate of all the other designs of the 1970s. However, it did incorporate some features that became almost standard in most modern prosthesis designs. The New Jersey, a cemented, two-component implant, consisted of a cylindrical surface ultrahigh-molecular-weight polyethylene (UHMWPE) talar component and a cobalt-chromium alloy tibial component, both with dual fixation fins.[45] The addition of a polyethylene meniscus in 1978 lead to the low contact stress (LCS) prosthesis, first implanted in 1981,[46] with survival rates of approximately 60% at 10 years. The LCS (evolved as the Buechel-Pappas [BP] prosthesis in 1984) was the first three-component total ankle replacement introducing the mobile-bearing joint replacement concept in ankle replacement.

Hakon Kofoed in 1978 introduced the initial Scandinavian Total Ankle Replacement (STAR) design. The first prosthesis was implanted in 1981, consisting of a metal talar component (covering the medial and lateral gutter talar surfaces), articulating with a polyethylene tibial component (two-component congruent unconstrained design). Both were fixed with polymethyl methacrylate cement. Results of this prosthesis revealed a 12-year survival rate of 70%.[47] This implant was modified later, becoming a three-component prosthesis, keeping its original name as the STAR prosthesis.

TOTAL ANKLE REPLACEMENT IMPLANTS: THE EVOLUTION

The prostheses of the "new era" started evolving in the early 1980s (see **Fig. 2**). Ankle arthroplasty implants of the first decade (1970s) were relatively constrained, consisting of two components one made of metal and one of polyethylene fixed with poly-methyl methacrylate cement (see **Fig. 1**). Because clinical results were far from satisfactory, newer designs were introduced. Differences between modern total ankle replacement implants exist. However, there is one fundamental modification, compared with the early era implants, namely the "meniscus," made of UHMWPE in most prostheses (with the exception of the TNK ceramic/metallic ankle arthroplasty).[16] In different implants the meniscus was either fixed with one of the metal implants of the tibia and talus, or was mobile. Thus, some prostheses, although consisting of three components (tibial, talar, and polyethylene), act as two-component implants. In the Agility, TNK, INBONE, Eclipse, and ESKA ankle implants, the meniscus is fixed to the tibial component and has no independent movement (fixed-bearing). However, other modern prostheses consist of three separate components (tibia, talus, mobile meniscus). Hence, modern total ankle replacement prostheses are classified as three-component versus two-component implants, and fixed-bearing and mobile-bearing implants.

The development of mobile-bearing implants was based on the concept that incongruent surfaces in constrained joint replacements lead to high local stresses and pressures, and therefore increase UHMWPE wear. Congruent surfaces, however, have the advantage that load is more evenly distributed across the surfaces. Mobile-bearing implants combine congruence with minimally constrained components to enable the soft tissues to control physiologic motion at the joint.[4,46,48]

Furthermore, polymethyl methacrylate cement fixation, which was common practice in the early era of total implant ankle replacement, was abandoned and newer-generation implants are inserted without polymethyl methacrylate cement. Improved biomaterials that enhance bone ongrowth and thus prosthesis fixation are being manufactured, and cementless fixation in total ankle replacement is the gold standard at present.[4,8,17,18]

Another parameter in the prosthesis design is the length of the tibial stem. BP-type implants (see **Fig. 1**) have adopted a relatively long tibial stem, requiring the tibial component to be inserted through an anterior tibial window. Other designers, based on the fact that the bone strength, especially at the distal tibia (and to a lesser extend in the talus), decreases below the surface and becomes less resistant to compressive loading, advocated the use of shorter pegs, rather than a stem. Kofoed, the designer of the STAR prosthesis (see **Fig. 1**), noted that only the most distal 1 to 1.5 cm of the tibia is solid subchondral bone: above this level, the bone marrow is loose and fatty, not suitable for implant fixation.[49] This applies to the design of the Agility, STAR, HINTEGRA, and BOX prostheses, which do not have a stem for tibial component fixation.[4]

TWO-COMPONENT ANKLE REPLACEMENT DESIGNS
Agility Total Ankle Replacement

The Agility (DePuy, Warsaw, IN) is the most widely published two-component implant, allowing space between the medial and lateral gutters to absorb rotational forces (the talar component can slide from side-to-side). Its implantation requires fusion of the syndesmosis (see **Fig. 1**), and this has proved to be a source of potential problems.[50] Furthermore, implantation of the Agility total ankle replacement requires more bone resection,[18] possibly compromising future revision options. In terms of ankle kinematics, this semiconstrained design does not replicate normal ankle motion, because the ankle slides from side-to-side during rotation and dorsiflexion and plantarflexion motion. It was the only Food and Drug Association (FDA)–approved ankle implant in the United States until 2006[4] and has been in continuous clinical use for more than 20 years. The designers of the implant published their results in 1998[51] and 2004[50] with a failure rate (revision or arthrodesis) of 6.6% in 686 cases from 1995 to 2004, compared with 11% in 132 total ankle replacements from 1984 to 1994.[50] Other surgeons[52–54] published less favorable outcomes. A recent systematic review of the literature revealed that 9.7% of 2312 ankle replacements had failed after a weighted mean follow-up of 22.8 months.[55] The failure rate was 15.8%, however, in 234 prostheses followed for longer (weighted mean of 6.6 years) in a systematic review published in 2010.[5]

INBONE Total Ankle System

The INBONE and INBOINE II Total Ankle Systems (Wright Medical technology, Arlington, TX), formerly known as the Topez Total Ankle Replacement System, has a relatively long modular intramedullary stem to allow tibial fixation. The stem consists of small, interconnecting pieces, and can be built-up piece-by-piece.[56] UHMWPE is fixed on the tibial tray. It received FDA approval in 2005. A recent publication presented the use of the INBONE prosthesis as a salvage procedure for revision to failed Agility total ankle replacements in five patients.[57] The long stem raises concerns regarding transmission of forces into the tibial metaphysis leading to loosening of the prosthesis.

Eclipse Total Ankle Replacement

The Eclipse (Integra LifeSciences, Plainsboro, NJ) was FDA approved in November 2006 but does not seem to be in regular clinical use in the United States. It can be implanted from a medial or lateral approach. The potential benefit is to avoid skin complications from an anterior approach; however, it can be complicated by malleolar nonunion or malunion.[17]

The TNK Prosthesis

Takakura introduced this prosthesis (Nara, Japan), fixed with or without cement, in Japan in 1975 (early version). The first- and second-generation implants were associated with high aseptic loosening rates, and biomaterials were modified. The third-generation (current) implant provided better outcomes.[16,58] The developers' team recommended cement talar component fixation in rheumatoid patients. Unfavorable clinical and radiographic outcomes in Japanese rheumatoid patients were reported in two studies.[59,60] It is currently the only total ankle replacement prosthesis with alumina ceramic components.

The ESKA Ankle Prosthesis

This two-component cementless prosthesis (polyethylene attached to the tibial component) was designed and used in Germany (ESKA, Lubeck, Germany), and is implanted through a lateral approach. Most foot and ankle specialists are more familiar with anterior ankle approaches and would not adopt the ESKA implant. According to the developer of the prosthesis, none of the implants followed for 1 to 5 years had failed; 17 (85%) of 20 total ankle replacements followed for 5 to 10 years were in situ, whereas 8 (67%) of 12 total ankle replacements remained in situ after 10 to 15 years.[61,62] No results from independent centers have been reported.

RAMSES Ankle Replacement

The RAMSES (Laboratoire Fournitures Hospitalieres, Heimsbrunn, France) was developed in 1989 in France by the Talus Group. They changed from using polymethyl methacrylate cemented implants (1989–2000) to cementless fixation since 2000. A 16.4% failure rate and a 61% radiolucency rate, after 10 to 14 years of follow-up in 73 ankles, using the polymethyl methacrylate cemented version, has been reported.[63] Concerns about the Ramses ankle implant are the wide talar bone resection, compromising future revision options, and the thin tibial loading platform (long-term fatigue possible).

THREE-COMPONENT (MOBILE-BEARING) ANKLE REPLACEMENT DESIGNS
BP-Type Designs

The BP prosthesis (see **Fig. 1**) (Endotec, Orange, NJ; and Wright-Cremascoli Orthopedics, a division of Wright Medical Technologies, Peschiera Borromeo, Italy), evolved from the LCS prosthesis in 1989[64] and was the predecessor of many modern implants (eg, the Mobility, Ankle Evolutive System, Zenith and CCI Evolution prosthesis).[4] It consists of three components (metal talus and tibia, separated by a mobile-bearing

UHMWPE "meniscus"), providing unconstrained motion with LCS on the bearing surfaces, allowing also inversion and eversion.[64] This prosthesis has further evolved in biomaterials and design. In their initial series of 40 total ankle replacements, the developers used a "shallow-sulcus" design, producing 70% good-to-excellent results after 2 to 20 years (mean, 12 years). A "deep-sulcus" design used in 75 ankles after 1990 revealed 88% good-to-excellent results after 2 to 12 years (mean, 5 years).[64] Doets and colleagues[65] reported 90% survivorship at 12 years in 74 BP (deep sulcus) implants, and San Giovanni and colleagues[66] reported 93.4% survivorship at 8 years. A review article reported an overall 12% failure rate after weighted mean follow-up of 6.3 years in 253 BP ankle replacements performed in several centers (including the developers' series).[4] Practically, the BP prosthesis is no longer marketed and has been replaced by its successors.

One concern regarding BP-type implants (implants having a tibial stem) is the need for an anterior tibial cortical window for insertion of the component, although it has not caused prosthesis failures according to the published studies. The main concern for tibial stems is that they rely for their fixation stability on the supramalleolar bone, which is loose and fatty and a less stable location to fix a prosthesis.[49,67] In the tibia and the talus, bone strength rapidly decreases below the surface, this being more apparent in the tibia, compared with the talus.[68]

The Mobility Total Ankle System

The Mobility Total Ankle System (De Puy, Warsaw, IN) is a more recently developed BP-type prosthesis, designed by a team of experienced ankle arthroplasty surgeons (Chris Coetzee in the United States, Pascal Rippstein in Switzerland, and Paul Wood in the United Kingdom). Unlike the BP prosthesis, the talar component of the Mobility Total Ankle System does not replace the medial and lateral surfaces of the talus. Two of the designers have published results from their own series. A failure rate of 2.1% in 233 arthroplasties, at a mean 33-months follow-up, with a postoperative complication rate of 8.6% and reoperation rate of 7.7%, was reported by Rippstein's and Coetzee's teams[69] and a 94.6% survivorship rate at 4 years by Wood.[70] Use of the prosthesis was documented in the New Zealand[23] and the Swedish Arthroplasty Registers.[19,20]

The Ankle Evolutive System

The Ankle Evolutive System (Biomet, Dordrecht, The Netherlands) is a cobalt-chromium three-component ankle prosthesis with hydroxyapatite coating, similar to the BP ankle prosthesis, but with some modifications (modular tibial stem, hemireplacement of the medial and lateral "gutters"). Given the high rates of aseptic loosening[71–74] it was withdrawn from the market.

Other BP-type prostheses are the Zenith (Corin, UK), designed by Winson (Bristol, UK)[75]; the German Ankle System (R-Innovation, Coburg, Germany), designed by Richter (Coburg, Germany)[76]; and the Alphanorm, designed by Tillman (Germany).[77] No results have been published yet for any of these designs. The CCI Evolution designed in the Netherlands and manufactured in Germany has a smaller tibial peg (compared with the BP).[78]

The STAR

The STAR (Waldmar Link, Hamburg, Germany; SBi, Morrisville, PA) (see **Fig. 1**) is at present one of the most widely used total ankle replacements. The first two-component STAR, metal-on-polyethylene cemented implant designed by Kofoed in 1978, was modified in 1986 when a mobile-bearing (meniscus) UHMWPE was introduced.[67] Two anchorage bars on the tibial component are meant to enhance fixation strength. The longitudinal ridge on the talar component is congruent with the distal surface of the mobile meniscus. The prosthesis allows dorsiflexion and plantarflexion, but no talar tilt, whereas the flat tibial surface of the meniscus allows rotation. Another modification was the bioactive surface coating for cementless fixation in 1990, and a double coating addition in 1999, to enhance bone ongrowth ability. Kofoed[49] reported a 95.4% survival rate for the uncemented design (1990–1995), which has not been reproduced by others.[5,19–21,79–84] Wood and colleagues reported in his series of 200 total ankle replacements an 80% survivorship at 10 years,[83] similar to Karantana and colleagues who found 84% survivorship at 8 years.[81] In a systematic literature review published in 2010, a 13% failure rate in 344 STAR implants, followed for a weighted mean of 6.3 years was reported.[5] A systematic review of published results on 2088 uncemented STAR prostheses revealed a pooled 71% survivorship rate at 10 years.[84] A Swedish group of surgeons[79,80] reported a 98% prosthesis survivorship at 5 years using 58 double-coated STAR prostheses, markedly better than the single-coated prosthesis used in earlier years.[80,81] Surgeons' experience influenced results.[20] The STAR is the first mobile-bearing, three-component ankle marketed in the United States. A recent publication of the first long-term STAR prosthesis survivorship data from the United States revealed a 90% survival rate at 10 years.[85] A potential issue with the STAR prosthesis is the lack of circumferential bone support of the tibial component, making it prone to sinking in the distal tibia cancellous bone, and possibly to periarticular ossification.[82,83]

HINTEGRA Total Ankle Arthroplasty

The HINTEGRA (Newdeal SA, Lyon, France) total ankle arthroplasty prosthesis, a three-component mobile-bearing implant (flat tibial component, UHMWPE meniscus, convex conic talus with a smaller medial radius), designed by Hinterman, has been in clinical use since 2000.[86,87] It relies on minimal bone resection to allow placement of the prosthesis in the very distal, better-quality cancellous subchondral bone. The talar and tibial components have ventral shields to allow screw placement, although the current trend is not to use screws for fixation because they could lead to loosening of the prosthesis during the initial phase of osteointegration. Side borders on the talar component should prevent dislocation of the polyethylene.[86,87] The anterior tibial flange aims to reduce postoperative heterotopic ossification and soft tissue adherence. The designer of the prosthesis reported a relatively high complication rate of 14% (39 complications in 278 implantations, and 13 failures) in his earlier case series (prostheses implanted before 2000), whereas the failure rate dropped after 2003. Overall survivorship in 340 primary total ankle replacements at 6 years was 98.2%, being 97.9% for the talar component and 98.8% for the tibial component.[86,87]

Salto Talaris Anatomic Ankle Prosthesis

The Salto (Tornier, Saint Ismer, France) is a newly designed version of the three-component mobile bearing implant, used in clinical practice since 1997 in Europe and approved for marketing by the FDA in 2006. It is fixed without polymethyl methacrylate cement, by a hollow fixation plug on the tibial side. Titanium plasma spray technology is used on the tibial and talar implants. The tibial surface of the UHMWPE is flat, and fits the congruent surface of the talar component with a sulcus, allowing varus-valgus motion in the coronal plane. Medial impingement is prevented by a medial metallic tibial rim, whereas a UHMWPE implant on the fibula replaces the talofibular joint.[88] Results from the developer's group in France show an 85%

survivorship at 8.9 years.[89] An independent series showed an estimated 87% 5-year survivorship.[90]

BOX Total Ankle Replacement

The BOX (Bologna-Oxford) total ankle replacement was designed after an Italian-British collaboration of the Rizzoli Orthopedic Institute, Bologna, Italy (Giannini, Catani, and Leardini) and Oxford University (O'Connor). The design rationale is to maintain complete congruency during the entire range of motion, to closely reproduce normal ankle kinematics.[15] A unique feature is that the mobile UHMWPE insert is concave on both sides (matching the convex tibial and talar components). It is fixed without polymethyl methacrylate cement. The tibial component is fixed with two parallel hollow bars, similar to the STAR prosthesis. Early results from nine centers show a 1.3% failure rate and a 4.4% reoperation rate in 158 ankles after mean follow-up of 17 months (range, 6–48-months).[91] Another study revealed a 92% survival rate in 62 ankles, after 42.5-months mean follow-up.[92]

HAVE THE INDICATIONS FOR TOTAL ANKLE REPLACEMENT CHANGED OVER THE YEARS?

Patient's selection is a fundamental issue to achieve good outcomes. Who is the ideal candidate for an ankle replacement, and what can be considered as contraindication to undertake an ankle replacement? For many surgeons, the best candidate is the relatively old patient with inflammatory arthropathy and multiple joint involvement with a stable, neutrally aligned ankle in the coronal plane.[93,94] The concept of the "well-aligned ankle in a rheumatoid elderly patient" is, however, largely debated.

There does not seem to be a clear age limit for total ankle replacement, with contrasting data from different studies. Published results from the 1990s showed that young patients do not do as well as older ones.[95] More recently published data from the same country (Sweden) revealed an increased risk of revision for patients with primary or posttraumatic osteoarthritis, younger than 60 years. This difference was statistically significant only for women, however, whereas the revision rate for rheumatoid patients was not influenced by age.[20] However, data from the Norwegian,[21] Finnish,[22] and New Zealand,[23] registers did not show higher revision rates for younger patients. However, higher demand and younger patients with higher activity levels may compromise the longevity of their total ankle replacement.

Individual surgeons have different approaches based on their familiarity with the procedure. Thus, some specialists expanded the indications performing total ankle replacement for more complex arthritic ankles, deformed more than 20 degrees in the coronal plane. Although malalignment has been considered a contraindication for total ankle replacement in the past,[4,8,9,93] it has been shown that is possible to perform a total ankle replacement, performing adjunctive procedures to correct alignment and stability (eg, subtalar or triple arthrodeses, calcaneal osteotomies, ligament reconstructions, malleolar osteotomies and osteoplasties).[94,96–98] These demanding procedures, which may increase the risk for complications, should be approached with caution, especially by inexperienced surgeons, because long-term outcome data are not available.

Patients with posttraumatic ankle osteoarthritis, the most frequent cause, may have less favorable outcomes because chronic instability or soft tissue contractures may compromise the outcome. Nevertheless, the range of motion after a total ankle replacement is not very different compared with the preoperative range of motion.[5] Therefore, it is questionable whether a very stiff arthritic ankle will benefit from a demanding total ankle replacement in terms of restoration of motion. The same applies for those patients who have an ankle fusion converted to total ankle replacement. A recent publication, however, revealed promising results in 29 fused ankles that were taken down to perform a total ankle replacement, followed for an average of 56 months (minimum, 3 years). The functional score improved significantly, only one total ankle replacement had to be revised, and 87% of patients were satisfied.[99] Less favorable, however, were the outcomes of a former publication, according to which of 23 ankles, four were lost to follow-up and 3 of the remaining 19 required a leg amputation.[100]

There is some recent evidence to suggest that obesity should not be a contraindication for total ankle replacement, because obese patients' outcomes are as good as those of patients with a normal body weight.[101] Indications for total ankle replacement have recently expanded to include certain patient groups (eg, those suffering from hemophilic arthropathy,[102] gout,[103] or hereditary hemochromatosis[104]) who may not have been considered as candidates for total ankle replacement in the past.[102–104] Paralytic conditions, such as poliomyelitis, were recognized as contraindications for total ankle replacement. However, a recent case report revealed expansion of the indications in these disorders.[105]

Evidence shows that surgeons attempted more often, in recent years, to salvage symptomatic total ankle replacements by revising one or some of the components. It depends on careful analysis and identification of the reasons for failure of the primary prosthesis. Outcomes of revision total ankle replacement are promising, with 6% aseptic loosening rate for 83 total ankle replacement revisions using the HINTEGRA prosthesis.[106] This may not only increase the number of revision total ankle replacements, but could also give surgeons the confidence to offer a primary total ankle replacement more easily, because a complex hindfoot fusion, associated with significant bone loss, is clearly not the only salvaging option if the total ankle replacement failed, for many patients.

Epidemiologic data show that the number of total ankle replacements procedures is increasing. The Swedish Joint Register showed that the annual number of total ankle replacements performed in Sweden progressively increased from 6 in 1993 to 74 in 2002, remaining steady at around 70 per year.[20] This indicated that one total ankle replacement per 100,000 inhabitants over the age of 15 is performed. This rate is the same in Norway[24] and Scotland[25] and is slightly higher in England and Wales, where it is 1.2.[26] Twice as many replacements are performed annually in Finland[22] and three times as many are performed in New Zealand[27] and Denmark (2.8 total ankle replacements per 100,000 inhabitants).[28] This is probably because advances in implant design, surgical techniques, and biomaterials lead to improved outcomes, and more surgeons feel confident to offer their patients the option of having a total ankle replacement instead of a fusion.

Presence of poor skin condition in the ankle region, tobacco use, peripheral vascular disease, or previous septic arthritis are conditions to be considered as possible contraindications for total ankle replacement because there is evidence of increased wound healing complication rate in these patients.[107] Similarly, other authors, reviewing a series of 106 total ankle replacements and applying multivariate regression analysis, found history of diabetes to be related to minor complications (wounds requiring only local care or oral antibiotics), whereas female gender, history of corticosteroid use, and underlying inflammatory arthritis were associated with major complications (requiring reoperation).[108] Active infection and Charcot neuro-osteo-arthropathy have been historically considered, and still are, absolute contraindications.[4,8,9,93,94]

ANKLE REPLACEMENT VERSUS FUSION

Ankle fusion was for decades the first choice in the management of end-stage ankle osteoarthritis, whereas total ankle replacements were scarcely performed. Currently, ankle fusion may still be the gold standard procedure to manage end-stage ankle osteoarthritis for most patients and most surgeons. However, total ankle replacement seems to have evolved to a viable alternative, at least for selected patents, with accumulating evidence of marked improvement in terms of the self-reported measures of impairments, quality of life, pain, and function, reported by patients.[109] A randomized trial showed that, at 24 months, ankles that received an STAR prosthesis had better function with equal pain relief compared with fused ankles.[110] Consistently, a systematic literature review published in 2007 revealed similar intermediate outcomes between ankle arthrodesis and total ankle replacement.[6] A comparative long-term outcome study would give more definite answers.

WHO SHOULD PERFORM A TOTAL ANKLE REPLACEMENT?

The importance of the learning curve has been highlighted in many published articles.[4,5,19,20] Outcomes reported from high-volume total ankle replacement surgeons, namely those who designed prostheses, are better regarding implant survivorship rates compared with studies from independent centers.[4,5] Whether this is related to bias, or is just the result of greater familiarity with the procedure, is debatable. Nevertheless, evidence from Sweden showed higher survivorship for the latter 31 ankle replacements surgeons performed (88% at 5 years and 65% at 10 years), compared with their first 20 (65% at 5 years and 37% at 10 years), all using the single coated STAR prosthesis.[80,81] Similarly, analysis of data from the Swedish joint register revealed improved survivorship of total ankle replacements, since small volume centers stopped performing these procedures.[20] Finally, a Korean study showed reduced perioperative complication rate after the first 25 total ankle replacements.[111] It seems that there is enough evidence to conclude that training and experience matter, and that total ankle replacements should be left for specialists familiar with primary implantation and revision techniques.

DISCUSSION

Primitive total ankle replacement designs used in the 1970s consistently failed[4] because surgeons had not recognized that the ankle is different compared with the knee and the hip joint. They had not taken into consideration the kinematics of the hindfoot joints, and did not predict the high stresses applied in the bone-implant interface when the ankle joint moves during gait.

In the early era of total ankle replacement, surgeons thought that because the ankle joint is highly congruent, constrained designs would provide better resistance to wear as a result of better pressure distribution. They did not appreciate the complex dynamic nature of the ankle axis of rotation[14] allowing complex triplanar motion (dorsiflexion/plantarflexion, eversion/inversion, internal rotation/external rotation).[12–14] They then realized that is was probably more important to restore compatible function of the ligaments and articular surfaces, using slightly nonanatomic shapes of the articular surfaces. Incongruent surfaces would, however, lead to high local stresses and pressures, and therefore increase UHMWPE wear. What could be the "golden mean" in total ankle replacement implant design to combine congruence and stability, with minimally constrained components allowing the ligaments to control physiologic motion at the ankle joint?

Three-component "mobile bearing" designs, initially used in knee replacement based on the LCS principle, were introduced in total ankle replacement to solve this problem. This key feature seems to represent a revolution in the history of total ankle replacement, and became the gold standard in Europe. In the United States, the STAR and BP implants have been used as part of clinical trials, and after the STAR prosthesis received FDA clearance in 2007[112] and the first long-term outcome report shows 90% survivorship at 10 years[86] although questions remain. The use of additional three-component mobile-bearing ankle prostheses may become first choice of implants in the United States.

Furthermore, polymethyl methacrylate cement fixation, which has long-term success in knee and hip implants, did not prove to be a good solution in the ankle. Polymethyl methacrylate cement fixation was, therefore, abandoned in the 1990s and efforts were made to enhance osteointegration and reduce contact stresses at the bone-implant interface. Practically all modern total ankle replacement implants have adopted a mobile-bearing, cementless fixation principle.

Although level I scientific evidence is not always available, the following issues have been clearly answered: nonconstrained, three-component, mobile-bearing implants reduce friction and polyethylene wear; cementless with bone ongrowth is superior to polymethyl methacrylate cement fixation; specialized centers and individual surgeons performing a high-volume of total ankle replacements provide superior outcomes; and survivorship of total ankle replacements is inferior to that of knee and hip replacements.

The latter shows that some hurdles are still in place, because total ankle replacements seem to be less successful compared with hip and knee replacements. The anatomic characteristics of the tibiotalar joint, with the reduced bone density of the distal tibia metaphysis,[47–49] the anatomy of the medial malleolus that makes it prone to fractures, the degeneration of the medial and lateral "gutters," the stiffness or ligament insufficiency in posttraumatic arthritic ankles, and the small size of the talus were factors that provided more challenges for the success of total ankle replacement, over the years. Some newer prostheses used improved implantation instrumentation to decrease bone resection and allow better bone quality for prosthesis fixation, and incorporated improved surface biomaterials.[4,17,18] Therefore, some designs moved away from stem tibial component fixation, using pegs, bars, or fins instead. This remains controversial. The same applies to the need for medial tibiotalar and tibiofibular joints replacement, because outcome studies do not provide definite conclusions.[4,5]

These are the factors that have limited long-term success of total ankle replacements over the years, so that it lies far behind that of hips and knees.[11] Because human ankle joint anatomy and function is not going to change, these factors may continue to limit attempts to improve the outcomes of ankle replacements, at least for difficult ankles and high-demand patients.

Nevertheless, history and evidence have shown that surgeons' expertise and experience matters. Also, patients' expectations have markedly changed over the years. Some patients would not accept surgery to their arthritic ankle as a salvage procedure, and required high-functional demands. Can an ankle replacement satisfy their needs and wishes? What should be considered as a contraindication? Has the definition of a contraindication changed over the years? Can the limits be pushed? The evidence is weak to support a universal acceptance of expansion of the indications. Careful monitoring of the evolution and auditing of outcomes in the long term is essential. High-quality evidence is needed to adopt novel techniques and new implants.

Despite increasing awareness and accumulated experience, total ankle replacement remains controversial in several aspects:

- Is total ankle replacement better than ankle fusion in the long term?
- Can the indications be expanded in deformed ankles? What is the limit?
- Is there a lower age limit?
- Is body weight a relative contraindication?
- Should patients participate in sports after total ankle replacement?
- Should total ankle replacements be attempted in previously fused ankles?
- Are neuromuscular and paralytic disorders an absolute contraindication?
- Which is the optimal solution after implant failure? Are revision total ankle replacements good enough?
- Is there an ideal implant design?
  - Are long tibial stems needed?
  - Is it necessary to replace the "gutters"?

Experimenting on patients based on "bright ideas" is definitely not the way forward. Studying the history helps clinicians succeed in the future. What went wrong and why? Do we have all the answers we need? Can clinicians improve outcomes and solve controversies? To achieve those targets, in the future:

- Surgeons, bioengineers, scientists should keep studying normal foot and ankle kinematics and try to produce implants that closely resemble it.
- Surgeons should identify the limitations, given that soft tissue balancing in the arthritic hindfoot is sometimes impossible.
- Level I long-term studies should provide high-quality evidence comparing total ankle replacements with ankle fusions.
- Systematic reviews and long-term cohort studies may provide useful conclusions, highlighting failures of certain implants/techniques.
- Technologic advances may enhance bone ongrowth onto the implant surfaces and reduce aseptic loosening rates.
- Improved instrumentation and surgical technique could improve accuracy of implantation and clinical outcomes.
- Patient selection was and remains a fundamental issue for success of total ankle replacements. Expansion of the indications by the average surgeon is only justified if high-level evidence is available.

SUMMARY

Time eliminated constrained, cemented, first-generation ankle replacements. Although some two-component, more anatomic, designs are still used, it seems that three-component mobile bearing ankle prostheses are winning the race of evolution. Not only have the implants changed over the years, but so have patients and surgeons. Surgeons specialize, improving their surgical outcomes and expanding the indications for total ankle replacement, in technically demanding, complex ankles. High-demand, younger patients, but also obese ones, are also potential candidates for a total ankle replacement. The future will set the limits, as enthusiasm over bright ideas was often followed by skepticism.

REFERENCES

1. Eloesser L. Implantation of joints. Cal State J Med 1913;11(12):485–91.
2. Muir DC, Amendola A, Saltzman CL. Forty-year outcome of ankle "cup" arthroplasty for post-traumatic arthritis. Iowa Orthop 2002;22:99–102.
3. Lord G, Marrotte JH. Total ankle replacement. Rev Chir Orthop Reparatrice Appar Mot 1980;66(8):527–30 [in French].

4. Gougoulias NE, Khanna A, Maffulli N. History and evolution in total ankle arthroplasty. Br Med Bull 2009;89:111–51.
5. Gougoulias N, Khanna A, Maffulli N. How successful are current ankle replacements? A systematic review of the literature. Clin Orthop Relat Res 2010;468(1): 199–208.
6. Haddad SL, Coetzee JC, Estok R, et al. Intermediate and long-term outcomes of total ankle arthroplasty and ankle arthrodesis. A systemic review of the literature. J Bone Joint Surg 2007;89:1899–905.
7. Coester LM, Saltzmann CL, Leupold J, et al. Long-term results following ankle arthrodesis for posttraumatic arthritis. J Bone Joint Surg 2001;83:219–28.
8. Guyer AJ, Richardson EG. Current concepts review: total ankle arthroplasty. Foot Ankle Int 2008;29(2):256–64.
9. Chou LB, Coughlin MT, Hansen S Jr, et al. Osteoarthritis of the ankle: the role of arthroplasty. J Am Acad Orthop Surg 2008;16(5):249–59.
10. Learmonth I, Young C, Rorebeck C. The operation of the century: total hip replacement. Lancet 2007;370:1508–19.
11. Labek G, Thaler M, Janda W, et al. Revision rates after total joint replacement: cumulative results from worldwide joint register datasets. J Bone Joint Surg Br 2011;93(3):293–7.
12. Deland JT, Morris GD, Sung IH. Biomechanics of the ankle joint. A perspective on total ankle replacement. Foot Ankle Clin 2000;5:747–59.
13. Siegler S, Chen J, Schneck CD. The three-dimensional kinematics and flexibility characteristics of the human ankle and subtalar joints. Part I. Kinematics. J Biomech Eng 1988;110:364–73.
14. Lundberg A, Svennson OK, Bylund C, et al. Kinematics of the ankle/foot complex. Part 3. Influence of the leg rotation. Foot Ankle 1989;9:304–9.
15. Leardini A, O'Connor JJ, Catani F, et al. Mobility of the human ankle and the design of total ankle replacement. Clin Orthop Relat Res 2004;424:39–46.
16. Takakura Y, Tanaka Y, Kumai T, et al. Ankle arthroplasty using three generations of metal and ceramic prostheses. Clin Orthop Relat Res 2004;424: 130–6.
17. Cracchiolo A III, Deorio JK. Design features of current total ankle replacements: implants and instrumentation. J Am Acad Orthop Surg 2008;16(9): 530–40.
18. Feldman MH, Rockwood J. Total ankle arthroplasty: a review of 11 current ankle implants. Clin Podiatr Med Surg 2004;21(3):393–406.
19. Henricson A, Skoog A, Carlsson A. The Swedish ankle arthroplasty register: an analysis of 531 arthroplasties between 1993 and 2005. Acta Orthop 2007;78(5):569–74.
20. Henricson A, Nilsson JÅ, Carlsson A. 10-year survival of total ankle arthroplasties: a report on 780 cases from the Swedish Ankle Register. Acta Orthop 2011; 82(6):655–9.
21. Fevang BT, Lie SA, Havelin LI, et al. 257 ankle arthroplasties performed in Norway between 1994 and 2005. Acta Orthop 2007;78(5):575–83.
22. Skyttä ET, Koivu H, Eskelinen A, et al. Total ankle replacement: a population-based study of 515 cases from the Finnish Arthroplasty Register. Acta Orthop 2010;81(1):114–8.
23. Hosman AH, Mason RB, Hobbs T, et al. A New Zealand national joint registry review of 202 total ankle replacements followed for up to 6 years. Acta Orthop 2007;78(5):584–91.
24. Available at: www.nrlweb.ihelse.net. Accessed January 6, 2012.
25. Available at: www.arthro.scot.nhs.uk. Accessed January 6, 2012.

26. Available at: www.njrcentre.org.uk. Accessed January 6, 2012.
27. Available at: www.cdhb.govt.nz. Accessed January 6, 2012.
28. Available at: www.sst.dk. Accessed January 6, 2012.
29. Buchholz HW, Engelbrecht E, Siegel A. Totale Sprunggelenks endoprothese Model St. George. Chirurg 1973;44:241–5.
30. Engelbrecht E. Ankle endoprosthesis model "St. George." Z Orthop Ihre Grenzgeb 1975;113:546–8 [in German].
31. Freeman MA, Kempson MA, Tuke MA. Total replacement of the ankle with the ICLH prosthesis. Int Orthop 1979;2:237–331.
32. Bolton-Maggs BG, Sudlow RA, Freeman MA. Total ankle arthroplasty. A long-term review of the London Hospital experience. J Bone Joint Surg 1985;67:785–90.
33. Waugh TR, Evanski PM, McMaster WC. Irvine ankle arthroplasty: prosthetic design and surgical technique. Clin Orthop 1976;114:180–4.
34. Evanski PH, Waugh TR. Management of arthritis of the ankle. An alternative of arthrodesis. Clin Orthop 1977;122:110–5.
35. Wynn AH, Wilde AH. Long-term follow up of the Conaxial (Beck-Steffee) total ankle arthroplasty. Foot Ankle 1992;3:303–6.
36. Stauffer RN, Segal NM. Total ankle arthroplasty: four years' experience. Clin Orthop 1981;160:217–21.
37. Kitaoka HB, Patzer GL, Strup DM, et al. Survivorship analysis of the Mayo total ankle arthroplasty. J Bone Joint Surg 1994;76:974–9.
38. Kitaoka HB, Patzer GL. Clinical results of the Mayo total ankle arthroplasty. J Bone Joint Surg 1996;78:1658–64.
39. Newton SE. Total ankle arthroplasty. Clinical study of fifty cases. J Bone Joint Surg 1982;64:104–11.
40. Kirkup J. Richard Smith ankle arthroplasty. J R Soc Med 1985;78:301–4.
41. Carlsson AS, Henricson A, Linde LR, et al. A 10-year survival analysis of 69 Bath and Wessex ankle replacements. Foot Ankle Surg 2001;71:39–44.
42. Jensen NC, Kroner K. Total ankle joint replacement: a clinical follow-up. Orthopedics 1992;15:236–9.
43. Schill S, Biehl C, Thabe H. Ankle prostheses. Mid-term results after Thompson-Richard sand STAR prostheses. Orthopade 1998;27:183–7 [in German].
44. Wood PL, Clough TM, Jari S. Comparison of two total ankle replacements. Foot Ankle Int 2000;21:546–50.
45. Pappas MJ, Buechel FF, DePalma AF. Cylindrical total ankle joint replacement: surgical and biomechanical rationale. Clin Orthop 1976;118:82–92.
46. Buechel FF, Pappas MJ, Iorio LJ. New Jersey low contact stress total ankle replacement: biomechanical rationale and review of 23 cementless cases. Foot Ankle 1988;8:279–90.
47. Kofoed H. Cylindrical cemented ankle arthroplasty. Foot Ankle Int 1995;16:474–9.
48. Hintermann B. Total ankle arthroplasty: historical overview, current concepts and future perspectives. New York: Springer – Wien; 2004.
49. Kofoed H. Scandinavian total ankle replacement (STAR). Clin Orthop Relat Res 2004;424:73–80.
50. Knecht SI, Estin M, Callaghan JJ, et al. The agility total ankle arthroplasty. Seven to sixteen-year follow-up. J Bone Joint Surg Am 2004;86:1161–71.
51. Pyevich MT, Saltzman CL, Callaghan JJ, et al. Total ankle arthroplasty: a unique design. Two to twelve-year follow-up. J Bone Joint Surg Am 1998;80:1410–20.
52. Hurowitz EJ, Gould JS, Fleising GS, et al. Outcome analysis of agility total ankle replacement with prior adjunctive procedures: two to six year follow up. Foot Ankle Int 2007;28(3):308–12.

53. Sprit AA, Assal M, Hansen ST Jr. Complications and failure after total ankle arthroplasty. J Bone Joint Surg 2004;86:1172–9.
54. Kopp FJ, Patel MM, Deland JT, et al. Total ankle arthroplasty with the agility prosthesis: clinical and radiographic evaluation. Foot Ankle Int 2006;27(2):97–103.
55. Roukis TS. Incidence of revision after primary implantation of the Agility™ total ankle replacement system: a systematic review. J Foot Ankle Surg 2012;51(2): 198–204.
56. Available at: http://www.inbone.com/DesignRationale.aspx/. Accessed January 06, 2012.
57. Devries JG, Berlet GC, Lee TH, et al. Revision total ankle replacement: an early look at agility to INBONE. Foot Ankle Spec 2011;4(4):235–44.
58. Tanaka Y, Takakura Y. The TNK ankle. Short- and mid-term results. Orthopade 2006;35:546–51 [in German].
59. Nishikawa M, Tomita T, Fujii M, et al. Total ankle replacement in rheumatoid arthritis. Int Orthop 2004;28:123–6.
60. Nagashima M, Takahashi H, Kakumoto S, et al. Total ankle arthroplasty for deformity of the foot in patients with rheumatoid arthritis using the TNK ankle system: clinical results of 21 cases. Mod Rheumatol 2004;14:48–53.
61. Rudigier J, Grundei H, Menzinger F. Prosthetic replacement of the ankle in post-traumatic arthrosis: 10-year experience with cementless ESKA ankle prosthesis. Eur J Trauma 2001;27:66–74.
62. Rudigier J, Grundei H, Menzinger F. Total ankle replacement: 14 year experience with the cementless ESKA ankle prothesis. Fuss Sprungg 2004;2:65–75.
63. Mendolia G, Coillard JY, Cermolacce C, et al, The Talus Group. Long-term (10 to 14 years) results of the ramses total ankle arthroplasty. Tech Foot Ankle Surg 2005;4(3):160–73.
64. Buechel FF Sr, Buechel FF Jr, Pappas MJ. Twenty-year evaluation of cementless mobile-bearing total ankle replacements. Clin Orthop Relat Res 2004;424:19–26.
65. Doets HC, Brand R, Nelissen RG. Total ankle arthroplasty in inflammatory joint disease with use of two mobile-bearing designs. J Bone Joint Surg 2006; 88(6):1272–84.
66. San Giovanni TP, Keblish DJ, Thomas WH, et al. Eight-year results of a minimally constrained total ankle arthroplasty. Foot Ankle Int 2006;27(6):418–26.
67. Kofoed H, Sorensen TS. Ankle arthroplasty for rheumatoid arthritis and osteoarthritis. J Bone Joint Surg 1998;80:328–32.
68. Hvid I, Rasmussen O, Jensen NC, et al. Trabecular bone strength profiles at the ankle joint. Clin Orthop 1985;199:306–12.
69. Rippstein PF, Huber M, Coetzee JC, et al. Total ankle replacement with use of a new three-component implant. J Bone Joint Surg Am 2011;93:1426–35.
70. Wood P, Karski M, Watmough P. Total ankle replacement. The results of 100 mobility total ankle replacements. J Bone Joint Surg Br 2010;92:958–62.
71. Kokkonen A, Ikävalko M, Tiihonen R, et al. High rate of osteolytic lesions in medium-term followup after the AES total ankle replacement. Foot Ankle Int 2011;32(2):168–75.
72. Henricson A, Knutson K, Lindahl J, et al. The AES total ankle replacement: a mid-term analysis of 93 cases. Foot Ankle Surg 2010;16(2):61–4.
73. Besse JL, Brito N, Lienhart C. Clinical evaluation and radiographic assessment of bone lysis of the AES total ankle replacement. Foot Ankle Int 2009;30(10):964–75.
74. Rodriguez D, Bevernage BD, Maldague P, et al. Medium term follow-up of the AES ankle prosthesis: high rate of asymptomatic osteolysis. Foot Ankle Surg 2010;16(2):54–60.

75. The ZENITH Total Ankle Replacement System. Available at: www.corin.co.uk. Accessed November 2, 2012.
76. Richter M, Zech S, Westphal R, et al. Robotic cadaver testing of a new total ankle prosthesis model (German Ankle System). Foot Ankle Int 2007;28(12): 1276–86.
77. Tillmann K. Endoprothetik am oberen Sprunggelenk. Orthopade 2003;32: 179–87 [in German].
78. Available at: www.vanstratenmedical.com. Accessed January 6, 2012.
79. Anderson T, Montgomery F, Carlsson A. Uncemented STAR total ankle prosthesis. J Bone Joint Surg 2003;85:321–9.
80. Carlsson A. Single- and double-coated star total ankle replacements: a clinical and radiographic follow-up study of 109 cases. Orthopade 2006;35(5):527–32 [in German].
81. Karantana A, Hobson S, Dhar S. The Scandinavian total ankle replacement: survivorship at 5 and 8 years comparable to other series. Clin Orthop Relat Res 2010;468(4):951–7.
82. Valderabano V, Hintermann B, Dick W. Scandinavian total ankle replacement. Clin Orthop Relat Res 2004;424:47–56.
83. Wood PL, Prem H, Sutton C. Total ankle replacement. Medium-term results in 200 Scandinavian total ankle replacements. J Bone Joint Surg Br 2008;90: 605–9.
84. Zhao H, Yang Y, Yu G, et al. A systematic review of outcome and failure rate of uncemented Scandinavian total ankle replacement. Int Orthop 2011;35(12): 1751–8.
85. Mann JA, Mann RA, Horton E. STAR™ ankle: long-term results. Foot Ankle Int 2011;32(5):473–84.
86. Hintermann B, Valderrabano V, Knupp M, et al. The HINTEGRA ankle: short- and mid-term results. Orthopade 2006;35(5):533–45 [in German].
87. Hintermann B, Valderrabano V, Dereymaeker G, et al. The HINTEGRA ankle: rationale and short-term results of 122 consecutive ankles. Clin Orthop Relat Res 2004;424:57–68.
88. Available at: http://www.tornier-us.com/lower/ankle/ankrec004/. Accessed January 6, 2012.
89. Bonnin M, Judet T, Colombier JA, et al. Midterm results of the salto total ankle prosthesis. Clin Orthop Relat Res 2004;424:6–18.
90. Schenk K, Lieske S, John M, et al. Prospective study of a cementless, mobile-bearing, third generation total ankle prosthesis. Foot Ankle Int 2011;32(8): 755–63.
91. Giannini S, Romagnoli M, O'Connor JJ, et al. Early clinical results of the BOX ankle replacement are satisfactory: a multicenter feasibility study of 158 ankles. J Foot Ankle Surg 2011;50(6):641–7.
92. Bianchi A, Martinelli N, Sartorelli E, et al. The Bologna-Oxford total ankle replacement: a mid-term follow-up study. J Bone Joint Surg Br 2012;94(6): 793–8.
93. Easley ME, Vertullo CJ, Urban WC, et al. Total ankle arthroplasty. J Am Acad Orthop Surg 2002;10(3):157–67.
94. Deorio JK, Easley ME. Total ankle arthroplasty. Instr Course Lect 2008;57: 383–413.
95. Kofoed H, Lundberg-Jensen A. Ankle arthroplasty in patients younger and older than 50 years: a prospective series with long-term follow-up. Foot Ankle Int 1999;20:501–6.

96. Knupp M, Bolliger L, Barg A, et al. Total ankle replacement for varus deformity. Orthopade 2011;40(11):964–70 [in German].
97. Mann HA, Filippi J, Myerson MS. Intra-articular opening medial tibial wedge osteotomy (plafond-plasty) for the treatment of intra-articular varus ankle arthritis and instability. Foot Ankle Int 2012;33(4):255–61.
98. Tan KJ, Myerson MS. Planning correction of the varus ankle deformity with ankle replacement. Foot Ankle Clin 2012;17(1):103–15.
99. Hintermann B, Barg A, Knupp M, et al. Conversion of painful ankle arthrodesis to total ankle arthroplasty. J Bone Joint Surg Am 2009;91(4):850–8.
100. Greisberg J, Assal M, Flueckiger G, et al. Takedown of ankle fusion and conversion to total ankle replacement. Clin Orthop Relat Res 2004;424:80–8.
101. Barg A, Knupp M, Anderson AE, et al. Total ankle replacement in obese patients: component stability, weight change, and functional outcome in 118 consecutive patients. Foot Ankle Int 2011;32(10):925–32.
102. Barg A, Elsner A, Hefti D, et al. Haemophilic arthropathy of the ankle treated by total ankle replacement: a case series. Haemophilia 2010;16(4):647–55.
103. Barg A, Knupp M, Kapron AL, et al. Total ankle replacement in patients with gouty arthritis. J Bone Joint Surg Am 2011;93(4):357–66.
104. Barg A, Elsner A, Hefti D, et al. Total ankle arthroplasty in patients with hereditary hemochromatosis. Clin Orthop Relat Res 2011;469(5):1427–35.
105. Morgan SS, Brook B, Harris NJ. Is there a role for total ankle replacement in polio patients? A case report and review of the literature. Foot Ankle Surg 2012;18(1):74–6.
106. Hintermann B, Barg A, Knupp M. Revision arthroplasty of the ankle joint. Orthopade 2011;40(11):1000–7 [in German].
107. Whalen JL, Spelsberg SC, Murray P. Wound breakdown after total ankle arthroplasty. Foot Ankle Int 2010;31:301–5.
108. Raikin SM, Kane J, Ciminiello ME. Risk factors for incision-healing complications following total ankle arthroplasty. J Bone Joint Surg Am 2010;92(12):2150–5.
109. Nunley JA, Caputo AM, Easley ME, et al. Intermediate to long-term outcomes of the STAR total ankle replacement: the patient perspective. J Bone Joint Surg Am 2012;94(1):43–8.
110. Saltzman CL, Mann RA, Ahrens JE, et al. Prospective controlled trial of STAR total ankle replacement versus ankle fusion: initial results. Foot Ankle Int 2009;30(7):579–96.
111. Lee KB, Cho SG, Hur CI, et al. Perioperative complications of HINTEGRA total ankle replacement: our initial 50 cases. Foot Ankle Int 2008;29(10):978–84.
112. US Food and Drug Administration Center for Devices and Radiological Health: Summary of the Orthopaedic and Rehabilitation Devices Panel Meeting – April 24, 2007. Available at: http://www.fda.gov/cdrh/panel/summary/ortho-04207.html. Accessed March 27, 2008.

Controversies in Total Ankle Replacement

Christopher Bibbo, DO, DPM, FACS, FACFAS

KEYWORDS

- Total ankle replacement • Bone-sparing implant • Ankle replacement guidelines
- Arthrodesis

KEY POINTS

- Total ankle replacement is in its infancy compared with other major joints.
- Traditional thinking regarding total ankle replacement (controversial issues) need to be scrutinized and reevaluated.
- There are both similarities and differences between total ankle replacement and hip/knee replacement, but "one shoe does not fit all."
- Indications for total ankle replacement are expanding.
- Much research still needs to be done to improve replacement techniques and the science behind designs for total ankle replacement.

INTRODUCTION

Total ankle replacement surgery is currently experiencing an unprecedented increase in use to treat symptomatic ankle-joint arthrosis. However, in comparison with hip and knee replacement, total ankle replacement is still on the steep slope of the learning curve not only for surgeons but also for applied ankle biomedical technology.

Hip and knee surgeons enjoy long-established sets of patient-selection criteria and extensive research on all outcomes of implant technology and patient outcomes. The ankle replacement surgeon, on the other hand, is still experiencing the "operate and learn" approach based on surgeon observations and experiences; truly, total ankle replacement is still in its infancy in comparison with hip and knee replacement. For those foot and ankle surgeons who are just starting to perform total ankle replacement, some helpful pearls are provided in **Box 1**.

Although there exist general guidelines regarding which patients are "suitable" candidates for total ankle replacement, these guidelines tend to be very conservative, much like those of knee and hip replacement from decades ago. There are also no head-to-head comparison studies of one total ankle replacement design versus

Foot & Ankle Section, Department of Orthopaedics, Marshfield Clinic, 1000 North Oak Avenue, Marshfield, WI 54449, USA
E-mail address: bibbo.christopher@marshfieldclinic.org

Clin Podiatr Med Surg 30 (2013) 21–34
http://dx.doi.org/10.1016/j.cpm.2012.08.003
0891-8422/13/$ – see front matter © 2013 Elsevier Inc. All rights reserved.

Box 1
Points to consider when embarking on total ankle replacement

- Plan every total ankle replacement with future revisions in mind.
- Select an implant system that makes "sense" to you, so that execution is intuitive to you.
- Never ignore preoperative malalignment.
- Be well versed in musculoskeletal disorders, especially in association with total ankle replacement.
- Avoid stress shielding.
- Avoid excessive bone resection.
- Do not accept suboptimal intraoperative results.
- Do not get in "over your head": total ankle replacement has a steep and long learning curve.
- Learn from your colleagues and follow sound joint-replacement and deformity correction principles.
- Scrutinize what industry brings to you: the latest or trendiest is not always the best.
- Start with straightforward cases; tackling complex cases and managing controversial issues should come with time and experience.

---

another. Because of the paucity of data, ankle surgeons are left to surmise the opinion based on limited studies, as well as (unfortunately) industry-sponsored data and the associated advertising material intended for sales and marketing of total ankle replacement devices. This article examines several key, controversial issues that apply to total ankle replacement. Recommendations and points for thought are based on the author's observations accrued over the past 15 years performing both upper extremity and lower extremity replacement surgery.

CONTROVERSIAL TOTAL ANKLE REPLACEMENT ISSUES
Is There Truly a Bone-Sparing Implant and is this Concept Really a Requirement?

Of the 4 total ankle replacement implants currently approved by the Food and Drug Administration (FDA) (STAR Ankle, Small Bone Innovations, Inc, Morrisville, PA; INBONE, Wright Medical Technology, Arlington, TN; Agility/Mobility, Depuy Orthopedics, Warsaw, IN; Salto Tolaris, Tornier, Edina, MN), all claim to some degree that their implant is bone sparing. Put very simply, whenever possible, while performing any replacement, preservation of natural bone and the architecture of opposing surfaces is desirable. As a surgeon who has had the privilege of performing major upper extremity, knee, and hip replacement surgery, the benefits of maintaining as much natural bone stock and joint mechanics has significant advantages both immediately and in the future if revision surgery is required. This school of thought has led to the introduction of hip resurfacing, which has revolutionized hip-joint surgery in younger patients. The author also believes that in the uncomplicated, primary arthritic ankle, without significant deformity, the implant of choice should mimic a joint-resurfacing procedure as much as possible; implantation proceeds via bone-sparing cuts. This problem is rather glaring with talar components that require large cuts, often resulting in subsidence of talar components, such as seen in the Agility total ankle replacement (**Fig. 1**). The current implant of choice that most closely mimics a joint resurfacing is the Salto Tolaris, which the author considers a first-line implant for uncomplicated total ankle replacement.

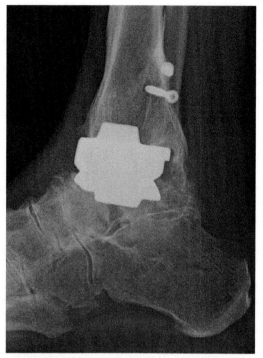

Fig. 1. Lateral radiograph demonstrating subsided, painful Agility talar component 5 years after surgery.

Take-home points

- Preserve bone and overall architecture on primary total ankle replacement.
- Think "joint resurfacing."
- Have a keen eye for preserving talar bone stock.
- Always think ahead: "how will my primary total ankle replacement affect any future revision efforts?"

Does a Total Ankle Replacement Need a Mobile Ultra–High Molecular Weight Polyethylene Insert?

Mobile-bearing elements were first introduced in knee replacement, with strong proponents of this design technology. The first total ankle replacement implant to successfully incorporate a mobile bearing was the Buechel-Pappas total ankle replacement (not FDA approved). It was the author's privilege to work with Dr Buechel (a clinician-scientist who was ahead of the curve) while in residency, which provided insight into the theory of mobile element design prosthesis, as well as getting to see first-hand his mobile-bearing knee and ankle (as well as early-design hip resurfacing) in action and in follow-up. Technical problems do exist with any mobile-bearing joint prosthesis, but the issues can be mitigated with proper design modifications. The European experience has witnessed a decline in mobile-bearing total ankle replacement, while in the United States the recent purchase of mobile-bearing designed implant (STAR Ankle) has led to a flurry of advertising, industry-sponsored "training" courses, and the occasional publication in the peer-reviewed literature. The real question is, "does the ankle truly require a mobile-bearing element?" The ankle, unlike the knee, is highly constrained, and experiences extreme concentrations of force across the joint. In the author's opinion, these factors lead to more shear on a mobile bearing within the ankle, resulting in significant 2-sided wear on the ultra–high molecular weight polyethylene (UHMWPE) insert, and a shifting of joint reactive forces and even excessive stress shielding. These problems have become evident with the STAR Ankle (**Fig. 2**), as well as reports of an unusually high 10% early failure rate requiring revision owing to difficulty with talar-component positions,[1] and a 5-year failure rate as high as 30%.[2]

Take-home points

- Ask yourself "does a mobile UHMWPE insert make sense to me?"
- Mobile bearings have track records of "spin-out," 2-sided wear and fracture.
- Are the short-term benefits worth the stress shielding/potential failure related to mobile bearing/implant design?

What About CT-Templated Patient-Specific Implants and "Navigation"?

Many experienced replacement surgeons will tell you that more often than not, patients are "betweens": the implant size for that patient falls between the sizes provided by industry-generated anthropometric measurements. Likewise, any experienced replacement surgeon will tell you that they can "operate" their way out of any difficulty they experience when suboptimal size disparities arise during surgery. So, where does the utility lie for an implant that matches a patient's specific anatomy based on computed tomography (CT) measurements submitted to the manufacturer? In knee replacement, contrary to what one may have surmised, this technique has not

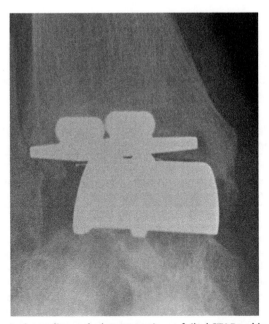

Fig. 2. Anterior-posterior radiograph demonstrating a failed STAR ankle replacement with ultra–high molecular weight polyethylene wear/fracture and stress shielding.

become the gold standard, not only for economic reasons but also for practical reasons; it is not of such benefit that existing techniques have become obsolete in comparison. However, as pointed out earlier, the ankle is vastly different to the knee; in cases where normal ankle anatomic landmarks are obscured and the position of natural joint line obliterated, a custom-fit implant may be a real rescue measure. The author has been involved in many cases where the contralateral "normal" side has had to be off-template to prevent overzealous talar resections as well as to preserve the medial malleolus, only to wish a custom implant was at hand. In these difficult cases where the usual architectural landmarks used to guide total ankle replacement bone resections are obscured, preoperative navigation with patient-specific implants and guides derived from contralateral CT measurements may prove to be of great assistance. At present, the only implant that allows patient-specific implants and navigation technology is the Prophecy INBONE Pre-Operative Navigation Alignment Guide for the INBONE total ankle replacement (released June 2012).

Take-home points

- Do not confuse true intraoperative navigation with preoperative "navigation"; the former produces patient-specific implants/jigs based on preoperative CT.
- Navigation-assisted replacement vis-à-vis preoperative CT-based templating is attractive on several levels, but currently is not proved to be superior to a well-executed standard total ankle replacement in primary total ankle replacement.
- Patient-specific implants may have the greatest value in complex cases and revisions, although they are not yet promoted for such cases.
- Intraoperative navigation is the next logical step; its value will need to be proved.

CONTROVERSIAL PATIENT ISSUES
Is the Varus and Valgus Extremity a Candidate for Total Ankle Replacement?

Although a very common topic of discussion, the seemingly controversial varus/valgus foot and ankle is a quite simple to approach: more work, but simple. First, a prosthetic joint needs to be placed in neutral on the frontal plane (as well as the sagittal plane), otherwise joint reactive forces accelerate implant failure.[3] When deformity exists, it needs to be broken down to the level of where the deformity occurs (eg, knee, tibia, supramalleolar, hindfoot, midfoot, and so forth), and the etiology of the deformity (eg, subsided old plateau fracture, tibial shaft or pilon malunions, posterior tibial tendon dysfunction, and so forth) (**Fig. 3**), and the deformity corrected at the appropriate anatomic/mechanical level or at an appropriate surrogate level (eg, calcaneal displacement osteotomy, Dwyer, Evans). Second, it must be remembered that with multilevel deformity, deformity correction starts proximally and continues distally (**Fig. 4**). Those unfamiliar with these concepts should not be performing total ankle replacement in patients with multilevel angular deformities. The same principles apply for the total ankle replacement patient with sagittal-plane deformity and limb-length inequality. Ligament, muscle, tendon, and osseous instability and deformity created by imbalance must be addressed before or simultaneously with total ankle replacement. It must also be stressed that navigation does not eliminate the need for a balanced mechanical axis (including the knee).

Take-home points

- Angular deformities (all planes) need to be corrected for total ankle replacement.
- Uncorrected angular deformity is a setup for failure of total ankle replacement.

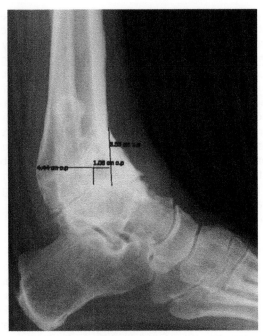

Fig. 3. Lateral radiograph of an 84-year-old male candidate for total ankle replacement with significant distal sagittal plane deformity and ankle arthrosis, best addressed by assigning a "new" joint line and using the INBONE total ankle replacement system.

- Small deformities (less than 10°) may be corrected with the INBONE total ankle replacement system; experienced surgeons may be able to solve smaller deformities with other total ankle replacement systems.
- Limb deformities that are multilevel (thigh, knee, ankle, foot) must have the most proximal deformity corrected first.
- Most often, deformity cases with ankle arthrosis that are candidates for total ankle replacement must be staged, starting proximally and ending distally with the total ankle replacement.

Diabetes, Neuromuscular Disorders, Steroid Use, Rheumatoid Arthritis, and Total Ankle Replacement?

One of the listed contraindications by the manufacturers of most total ankle replacement systems is neuromuscular disease. Unfortunately, a wide net has been thrown by this listing, excluding many patients who could have otherwise benefited from total ankle replacement. The surgeon is the ultimate judge of who is or is not a candidate for total ankle replacement, and must be well versed in the natural history of neuromuscular disorders, whether acquired or inherited, and understand the consequences of such disorders on joint mechanics and on the overall functional capacity of the patient with such afflictions. For example, poststroke patients, who have reached their plateau in recovery, may be candidates for total ankle replacement accompanied with appropriate tendon transfers.[4] The surgeon must also be very knowledgable on the systemic effects of disease states. For example, diabetes is not a contraindication to hip a knee replacement, nor is it for total ankle replacement, unless significant neuropathy is present or a Charcot process is present. The author carefully stratifies

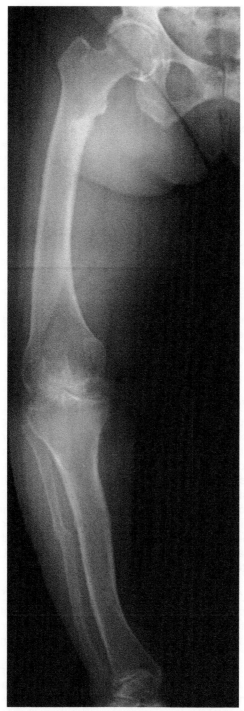

Fig. 4. Full-leg radiograph of a patient with hypophosphatemic rickets with disabling hip, knee, and ankle pain. Sequentially the hip, knee, distal tibia, then the ankle need to be addressed.

diabetic patients into insulin-dependent and non–insulin-dependent, followed by a 12-month analysis of hemoglobin A1c and degree of peripheral sensorimotor neuropathy.

Steroid use is listed as a relative contraindication for total ankle replacement; however, the key issue is bone stock. There is no uniformly accepted bone-density value for the ankle for which total ankle replacement is acceptable; thus, the clinician must rely on plain radiographic appearance. If there is any question, the author will obtain a CT to look for occult cysts in the talus and distal tibia that may require bone grafting and/or "temporary" cementation during total ankle replacement; one can never be too prepared for these difficult cases. Similarly, the author does not find the need to withhold antirheumatoid medications in the perioperative period, especially if withholding medications results in disabling rheumatoid flares that hinder physical therapy and rehabilitation efforts.[5–8] Postoperative management plans (weight bearing and so forth) must be individualized in such patients.

Take-home points

- Various neuromuscular disorders may be amenable to total ankle replacement, but require very careful thought and meticulous planning.
- Diabetes per se is not a contraindication to total ankle replacement; however, Charcot neuro-osteoarthropathy is!
- Corticosteroids adversely influence bone stock, but total ankle replacement may still be performed in properly selected patients.
- Rheumatoid arthritis is not a contraindication to total ankle replacement; however, these patients require significant preoperative planning and special techniques to ensure a secure, stable implant.
- Postoperative weight bearing and physical therapy programs must be individualized in these fragile patients.

Is Young Age a Contraindication to Total Ankle Replacement?

Traditionally joint replacement has been relegated to the elderly patient. Recent innovations and advances have propelled both knee and hip replacement indications to include younger patients. Likewise, the author, analyzing his own unpublished data, has found a significant role for total ankle replacement in young(er) patients, with good short-term results. In younger patients, extensive preoperative and postoperative counseling must stress that all total ankle replacements are designed for activities of daily living and not for sports, heavy lifting, jumping, running, and so forth. Patients must be well informed that revision is likely, and that catastrophic failure may occur quickly if strict adherence to activity limits are not followed. In the event of failure, each patient's management plan must be individualized; surgical interventions must not hinder future interventions 2 to 3 decades further on in life.

Infection and Total Ankle Replacement Reimplantation After Infection?

The bane of all musculoskeletal surgeons is infection, especially osteomyelitis in association with an injected joint prosthesis. The topic of the infected prosthetic joint can fill an entire issue of *Clinics*, but an attempt is made here at condensing the topic into several key points.

The infected joint replacement takes on many facets; the workup and management is complex and still riddled with many questions. The reported rates of infection after total ankle replacement vary widely and are not well defined, likely influenced by level of complexity, position of the learning curve, and individual definitions of infection. Published infection rates are as follows. STAR Ankle: superficial 1.2%, deep 1.2%[9]; Agility: 2.4% to 14%[10,11]; Salto Tolaris: no data published specific to infection rates at the time of this writing; INBONE: no data published specific to infection rates at the time of this writing. Clearly much work needs to be done in the area of managing the infected total ankle replacement.

So to date there is a paucity of data on how to best manage total ankle replacement infections. Taking a page from hip and knee replacement, as well as the author's extensive experience in managing complicated musculoskeletal infections for over 15 years, one can arrive at several principles: if it acts like an infection, treat it as such—be suspicious; early nonaggressive infections may be treated with retention of the implant; delayed infections (>8 weeks) are associated with biofilm formation and may require explantation, with UHMWPE insert removal at a minimum. Traditional cell counts are open to subjective interpretation and sampling error. Do not rely on cell counts alone; aerobe, anaerobe, fungal cultures, and 16S ribosomal DNA polymerase chain reaction analysis (16S PCR) are now the minimum standard for evaluating potentially infected prosthetic joint fluid, peri-implant issues, and explanted implants. In addition, following the lead of investigators at the Mayo Clinic and others[12,13] at explantation, the author sonicates the explanted total ankle replacement and cultures the sonicate to improve culture yields, which is especially useful in patients with subclinical infections and those who have received a recent course of antibiotics. In analyzing the author's unpublished data, not only are occult pathogens being uncovered but also bacterial species previously not recognized as part of the biofilm community in human implants. In managing the infected total ankle replacement, it cannot be overstressed to not "burn bridges": always consider how you may be affecting future reconstructive efforts (**Fig. 5**). Some basic guidelines when facing the infected total ankle replacement are listed here.

Author's workup of the infected total ankle replacement

Culture Modalities on All Suspected Infected Total Ankle Replacements:

- Laboratory tests: baseline erythrocyte sedimentation rate (ESR), C-reactive protein (CRP), complete blood cell count; serial labs during treatment (calcitonin levels are not reliable in the author's experience)

- Aerobe, anaerobe, acid fast, fungal; hold negative cultures for specimen for 16S PCR; 18S PCR for all fungal growth not identifiable by standard fungal culture techniques

- Intraoperative Gram stain; cell count? (not reliable)

- Culture modalities on tissue, and implant

- Sonicate implant and culture

Have a regimented approach to treating infected total ankle replacements

---

Surgical protocols for the infected total ankle replacement

UHMWPE Insert Exchange:

- Early infection of less than 4 weeks with nonresistant (sensitive) organisms

- (+) bone ingrowth of implant:

- Irrigation and débridement, exchange poly, culture-specific parenteral antibiotics 6 to 8 weeks

---

Staged Implant Salvage:

- Infection longer than 6 to 8 weeks, or early infections with resistant organisms and tissue destruction, aggressive fungal infections (eg, mucormycosis)
- Radical irrigation and débridement, culture
- Antibiotic spacer: at least 2 antibiotics; high levels (eg, 2–4 g vancomycin plus 4–6 g aminoglycoside per 20–40 g polymethylmethacrylate cement)
- Culture-specific antibiotics 6 to 8 weeks; aspiration or joint tissue (preferred)
- Cultures off antibiotics for 2 weeks; repeat all culture modalities; no reimplant unless all culture modalities are negative
- Replant?: After 8 weeks parenteral antibiotics, surgical culture modalities are (−) with patient off antibiotics for 2 weeks, normalized ESR and CRP
- Suppressive long-term oral antibiotics? (consult with infectious disease specialist)

The reconstruction

Postinfection Reconstruction Pearls

- Obtain CT to determine the quality and architecture of bone for feasibility of revision total ankle replacement after infection
- Fully evaluate the soft-tissue envelope: can it withstand surgical approach/healing again? Has there been a change in the patient's vascularity?
- Try not to remove the fibula at irrigation and débridement(s): limits later reconstructions to fusion only; may make fusion more difficult; lateral skin/wound issues are common after lateral approach and fibula resection
- Consider the patient's overall health and functional capacity to enjoy total ankle replacement reimplantation
- First- and second-degree arthrodesis: good options, especially with fine-wire circular external fixation
- Amputation is a very last resort but must not be forgotten as a therapeutic option

Take-home points

- Any signs or symptoms of infection must be fully evaluated ("if it walks like a duck, talks like a duck...").
- If a single infection criterion is met (eg, elevated ESR or CRP, redness with swelling, night pain, and so forth), the patient requires a full workup and is to be treated as an infected replacement until microbiologically proved otherwise.
- Subclinical infections are more common than previously recognized.
- Do not rely on cell counts; anaerobe, aerobe, fungal cultures, and 16S PCR are mandatory.
- Treatment of prosthetic joint infections requires an experienced multidisciplinary team.
- Reconstructive options after deep infections include reimplantation (limited data) and fusion; amputation is rarely required unless associated with massive tissue loss.

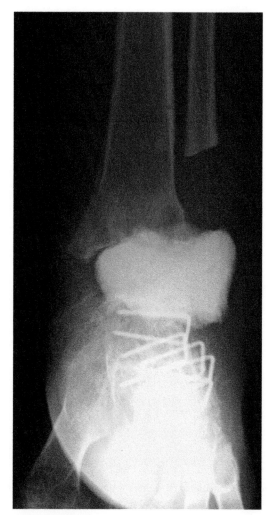

Fig. 5. Anterior-posterior radiograph demonstrating an antibiotic loaded polymethylmethacrylate cement spacer for deep infection after total ankle replacement. Note that the fibular resection may hinder future reconstructive efforts.

The Poor Anterior Soft-Tissue Envelope: Abandon Total Ankle Replacement Versus Modified Anterior Incision? Posterior Approach?

One near absolute contraindication for total ankle replacement, besides adequate arterial inflow to support bone and skin healing, is an anterior soft-tissue envelope that is incapable of supporting the standard anterior approach to the ankle. Free tissue and local tissue transfer is a salvage option for wound-healing issues, but is not acceptable to plan as a procedure done in conjunction with total ankle replacement at the time of a primary index operation. To circumnavigate the hostile anterior soft-tissue envelope of the ankle, the author has used two techniques. The first technique is to use a modified anterior approach (anterior Bibbo approach) that elevates a full-thickness flap of tissue, preserving any remaining ankle skin–perforating vessels (**Fig. 6**). This anterior incision preserves the anterior ankle skin perforators, and

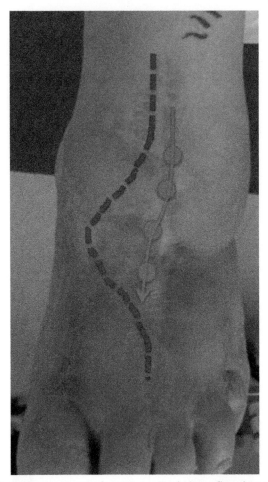

Fig. 6. The modified anterior approach creates a single-layer flap that spares the anterior tibial artery and perforators.

elevates the anterior soft-tissue envelope as one thick composite layer, further avoiding separation of scarred layers that may otherwise injure fragile skin perforators.

Truly controversial is the posterior approach to the ankle for total ankle replacement. Although recently popular for internal fixation of pilon fractures,[14] ankle/hindfoot fusions,[15] and oncology cases,[16] the posterior approach for execution of total ankle replacement (posterior Bibbo approach) (**Fig. 7**) has been described by the author (C. Bibbo, unpublished data). This posterior approach has also been performed successfully by James K. DeOrio, MD and Thomas Lee, MD with initial early success (personal communication, 2012). The posterior approach may find more utility in the future, but for now it is recommended only in extreme circumstances by experienced surgeons.

Take-home points

- In general, a hostile anterior soft-tissue envelope is a strong relative contraindication to total ankle replacement.

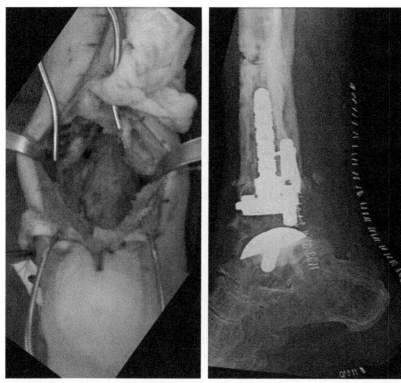

Fig. 7. Intraoperative photograph demonstrating the posterior approach for insertion of an INBONE total ankle replacement (demonstrated in immediate postoperative radiograph on the right). Note that the components have been placed "backward" in the ankle owing to the posterior approach.

- Thoroughly evaluate the healing potential of the patient by history, physical examination, and noninvasive arterial studies; refer for vascular surgery evaluation if there is any uncertainty.
- The modified anterior incision may be valuable in the hands of surgeons who understand the perforator anatomy of the leg and ankle.
- The posterior approach for total ankle replacement should only be attempted in extreme circumstances by the experienced replacement surgeon.
- Be versed in wound and plastic surgery techniques for incisions in the event of wound breakdown.

SUMMARY

The author provides multiple take-home points and pearls for performing total ankle replacement surgery, as well as situations whereby failure can be predicted and therefore total ankle replacement avoided. Surgeon adherence to the time-tested principles of total joint replacement is paramount to a successful outcome. Alternative approaches and novel techniques are available, but should be performed by those experienced in complex total ankle replacement.

REFERENCES

1. Dhawan R, Turner J, Sharma V, et al. Tri-component, mobile-bearing, total ankle replacement—mid-term functional outcome and survival. J Foot Ankle Surg 2012 Sep;51(5):566–9. Available at: http://www.ncbi.nlm.nih.gov/pubmed/22770902.
2. Anderson T, Montgomery F, Carlsson A. Uncemented STAR total ankle prostheses. Three to eight-year follow-up of fifty-one consecutive ankles. J Bone Joint Surg Am 2003;85(7):1321–9.
3. Espinosa N, Walti M, Favre P, et al. Misalignment of total ankle components can induce high joint contact pressures. J Bone Joint Surg Am 2010;92(5):1179–87.
4. Bibbo C, Baronofsky HJ, Jaffe L. Combined total ankle replacement and modified bridle tendon transfer for end-stage ankle joint arthrosis with paralytic dropfoot: report of an unusual case. J Foot Ankle Surg 2011;50:453–7.
5. Bibbo C. Wound healing complications and infection following surgery for rheumatoid arthritis. Foot Ankle Clin 2007;12:509–24.
6. Bibbo C. The assessment and perioperative management of patients with rheumatoid arthritis. Tech Foot Ankle Surg 2004;3:126–35.
7. Bibbo C, Goldberg JW. Infectious and healing complications after elective orthopaedic foot and ankle surgery during tumor necrosis factor-alpha inhibition therapy. Foot Ankle Int 2004;25:331–5.
8. Bibbo C, Anderson RB, Davis WH, et al. Complications in rheumatoid foot and ankle reconstructive surgery: analysis of 718 procedures in 103 patients. Foot Ankle Int 2003;24:40–4.
9. Saltzman CL, Mann RA, Ahrens JE, et al. Prospective controlled trial of STAR total ankle replacement versus ankle fusion: initial results. Foot Ankle Int 2009;30:579–96.
10. Spirit AA, Assal M, Hansen ST Jr. Complications and failure after total ankle arthroplasty. J Bone Joint Surg Am 2004;86:1172–8.
11. Claridge RJ, Sagherian BH. Intermediate term outcome of Agility ankle arthroplasty. Foot Ankle Int 2009;30:824–35.
12. Trampuz A, Piper KE, Jacobson MJ, et al. Sonication of removed hip and knee prostheses for diagnosis of infection. N Engl J Med 2007;357:654–63.
13. Holinka J, Bauer L, Hirschl AM, et al. Sonication cultures of explanted components as an add-on test to routinely conducted microbiological diagnostics improve pathogen detection. J Orthop Res 2011;29:617–22.
14. Ketz J, Sanders R. Staged posterior tibial plating for the treatment of orthopaedic trauma association 43C2 and 43C3 tibial pilon fractures. J Orthop Trauma 2012;26:341–7.
15. Nickisch F, Avilucea FR, Beals T, et al. Open posterior approach for tibiotalar arthrodesis. Foot Ankle Clin 2011;16:103–14.
16. Maheshwari AV, Walters JA, Henshaw RM. Extensile posterior approach to the ankle with detachment of the Achilles tendon for oncologic indications. Foot Ankle Int 2012;33(5):430–5.

Techniques for Managing Varus and Valgus Malalignment During Total Ankle Replacement

Woo Jin Choi, MD, Hang Seob Yoon, MD, Jin Woo Lee, MD, PhD*

KEYWORDS

- Total ankle replacement • Ligament balancing • Peri-talar instability

KEY POINTS

- One of the most critical determinants of long-term total ankle replacement survival is soft-tissue balancing.
- Superimposed degenerative change and deformity affecting the neighboring joints adds another level of complexity to the soft-tissue balancing equation.
- It is important that surgeons be provided with a rationale and a technique for the sequence of release and additional procedures commonly performed in balancing varus and valgus ankle in primary total ankle replacement.

Total ankle replacement has emerged as a promising alternative to ankle arthrodesis, the standard operation for the relief of pain owing to advanced osteoarthritis of the ankle, with favorable clinical results, high rates of patient satisfaction, and improved survivorship.[1–5] Successful total ankle replacement depends on many factors, including patient selection, prosthetic component design, alignment, ligament stability, and rehabilitation. Attention to all of these details is required to maximize outcomes and patient satisfaction. One of the most critical determinants of long-term implant survival is soft-tissue balancing; residual angular deformity or instability can lead to progressive edge loading, subluxation of the ultra-high molecular weight polyethylene (UHMWPE) insert, and premature failure.[6,7] Several authors have suggested that increased preoperative frontal plane deformity negatively influences the long-term results of total ankle replacement, and that ankle varus or valgus of more than 10° to 15° is a relative contraindication to total ankle replacement.[6–11] More recently, however, a variety of corrective procedures have been introduced to address soft-tissue imbalance and bony deformity, and satisfactory short-term results have been reported.[12–14]

Department of Orthopaedic Surgery, Yonsei University College of Medicine, 50 Yonsei-ro, Seodaemun-gu, Seoul 120-752, South Korea
* Corresponding author.
E-mail address: ljwos@yuhs.ac

Clin Podiatr Med Surg 30 (2013) 35–46
http://dx.doi.org/10.1016/j.cpm.2012.08.004
0891-8422/13/$ – see front matter © 2013 Elsevier Inc. All rights reserved.

In most end-stage arthritic ankles, some degree of instability, deformity, contracture, or combination of these elements is found.[6–10,12,13] Deformity and instability can stem from asymmetric loss of articular cartilage resulting in ligamentous, capsular, and musculotendinous imbalance. Contracture of soft tissues is a secondary change that generally arises as a consequence of trauma or long-standing angular malalignment. In general, medial-lateral soft-tissue balancing requires release of contracted soft tissue on the concave side of the deformed ankle. Release of contracted medial soft tissue in varus ankles is, for the most part, quite different from release of contracted lateral structures in valgus ankles. Superimposed degenerative change and deformity affecting the neighboring joints adds another level of complexity to the soft-tissue balancing equation.[14–17] Even if bone cuts can be made to establish anatomic alignment, proper soft-tissue balance is required to maintain alignment throughout the range of motion. It is important, therefore, that surgeons be provided with a rational thought process and predictable techniques to perform soft-tissue release and additional procedures commonly performed in balancing varus and valgus ankle in primary total ankle replacement. Although implant designs can vary considerably, the principles of ligament balancing are consistent. The approach we describe here is based on anatomic studies, clinical outcomes, and the authors' clinical experience.

OPERATIVE TECHNIQUE
Preoperative Planning

Although patient selection is possibly the single most important factor to achieving successful results after total ankle replacement, indications for total ankle replacement are still being defined. The optimal patient is older with end-stage arthritis, and nonobese and with low physical demands. A comprehensive musculoskeletal examination should be undertaken. This examination should include determination of potential sources of referred pain as well as local examination of the ankle. The contralateral ankle, both knees, and feet should be examined. In addition, inadequate vascularity or sensibility should be investigated thoroughly before total ankle replacement is considered. Standard preoperative radiographs should include standing anteroposterior and lateral views of the ankle, hindfoot alignment views, and long bone lower extremities views. Varus and valgus stress views are also necessary to evaluate the degree of instability and the reducibility of the deformity. Weight bearing anteroposterior and lateral views of foot should also be taken to check the presence of degenerative changes in adjacent joints, such as the subtalar and midtarsal joints. Magnetic resonance imaging can help to determine the cause of symptoms when associated soft-tissue pathology is suspected and to plan appropriate treatment thereof.

It is necessary to thoroughly evaluate malalignment and instability during preoperative planning. Both can result in subluxation and edge-loading of the UHMWPE insert, progressive deformity, and high early failure rates.[6–10,18] There is, however, controversy regarding the appropriate management strategies of varus or valgus deformity. Most authors agree that there are limits to the correction of varus or valgus deformity, and a deformity more than 20° is suggested as a contraindication to total ankle replacement.[19,20] If the frontal plane deformity is less than 10° or 15°, the indication for total ankle replacement should not be questioned. However, as mentioned, some authors stressed narrowing this indication to less than 10°,[7,15] whereas other investigators did not find significant differences between a group of patients with frontal plane deformity up to 10° and a second group with deformity greater than

10°.[12–14] Therefore, rather than establishing definite criteria, the authors believe that it is more appropriate for the surgeon to be aware of their ability to thoroughly correct all problems.

In the frontal plane, the degree of alignment of the ankle is formed by the anatomic axis of the tibia and a line perpendicular to the articular surface of the dome of the talus on a standing anteroposterior radiograph.[6,21] For angle alignments of less than 10° of varus or valgus, the joint is thought to be neutral, and considered to be varus or valgus when more than 10°.[6] Talar tilt angle is defined by the tibial and talar articular surfaces of the ankle joint on a standing anteroposterior radiograph.[7] For talar tilt angles of greater than 10°, the joint is defined as incongruent.[7] Deformities can be located at the joint level (usually owing to anatomic joint line malalignment or to ankle degeneration) or proximally (usually owing to tibial fracture).[22] If an abnormal alignment of more than 10° in any plane is present above the level of the ankle joint, corrective osteotomy must be performed at the level of deformity before total ankle replacement.[15,16,19,23] If the deformity of the ankle is located at the joint level, we recommend an algorithmic approach to soft-tissue balancing in varus ankles, including gradual release of the medial deltoid ligament, along with additional procedures (**Fig. 1**).[13,14]

Operative Procedure

Medial release and gap balancing
Ligament balance is achieved by progressively releasing medial soft tissue until they reach the length of lateral ligamentous structures. The extent of the release can be monitored by periodically inserting lamina spreaders or using a ligamentous tension meter to gauge alignment. Alternatively, trial components can be inserted, taking the ankle through by applying varus and valgus stress to the ankle.

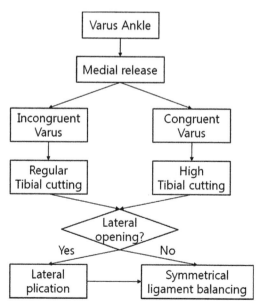

Fig. 1. Treatment algorithm and ligament balancing in varus ankle osteoarthritis. After sufficient medial release, the level of neutralizing tibial osteotomy is determined depending on the congruency of the varus. Any lateral laxity or instability with varus stress requires a lateral ligament plication procedure.

After the operative approach and ankle joint exposure, removal of peri-articular osteophytes from the distal tibia and talus can be performed to effectively lengthen medial capsuloligamentous tissue. Posterior osteophytes of the distal tibia should be carefully removed because they can lead to heterotopic ossification[24] or restrict the sagittal plane range of motion of the ankle. The next step in soft-tissue balancing involves correction of any talar tilt before making bone cuts. Gradual release of the deltoid ligament should be performed at its distal insertion using a curved osteotome. It is important to release all components of the deep deltoid ligament: The anterior tibiotalar, tibionavicular, and posterior tibiotalar ligaments. This gradual releasing was developed to alleviate the risk of medial ligamentous instability (or osteonecrosis of the talus) after extensive stripping from the talus, and to optimize ligamentous balancing. After bone preparation, trial components are then placed and varus and valgus stress is applied to the ankle to assess balancing. The ankle is inspected for residual medial tightness or lateral gapping in a neutral position. In ankles with moderate to severe varus, the medial compartment of the ankle commonly remains tighter than the lateral compartment. A more definitive medial release should be performed at this time to balance the ankle. Once all the extra-articular deformities are noted, such as tightness in the posterior tibial tendon, patients require another incision to release the relevant contracture.

Lateral plication-peroneus longus transfer to peroneus brevis

Any residual imbalance in the supine position can result in subluxation or dislocation of the UHMWPE insert component on weight-bearing. Several authors have shown that when the UHMWPE insert laterally subluxes with moderate varus stress or lateral opening is observed without applying any stress lateral plication can be performed through several techniques: Anatomic or nonanatomic lateral ligament reconstruction and bony procedures.[13,14,19] We prefer a modified Broström procedure[25] when the lateral ligamentous complex is spared (**Fig. 2**). In patients with long-standing varus ankle arthrosis, however, varus deformity is commonly associated, to some extent, with chronic lateral ankle instability. Varus deformity is frequently associated with loss of the anterior talofibular ligament and calcaneofibular ligament, as well as anteriorly displaced talus. In such cases, several nonanatomic reconstruction procedures can be performed. The authors have achieved satisfactory results with a peroneus longus tendon transfer to the base of the fifth metatarsal,[13] as described by Kilger et al.[26] This procedure effectively enhances lateral ankle stability and weakens plantar flexion force over the first metatarsal. In addition, it is easy to combine with Total Ankle Replacement (TAR). To perform this procedure, a small, longitudinal incision is made over the base of the fifth metatarsal. The sural nerve and small saphenous vein course just posterior to the tendon and are subcutaneous at this level. The peroneus brevis insertion to the base of the fifth metatarsal is observed and the peroneus longus is identified adjacent to the peroneus brevis tendon. The peroneus longus tendon is transected at its most distal portion in full plantar flexion and eversion of the ankle to allow for sufficient harvesting of the tendon. A suture anchor can be used at the base of the fifth metatarsal, just plantar and lateral to the insertion of the peroneus brevis tendon. The peroneus longus tendon is sutured under moderate tension while the foot is held in a slightly plantarflexed and everted position. This helps to provide sufficient eversion power postoperatively. A side-to-side tenodesis is then performed between the residual peroneus longus and brevis tendons. Degeneration or attritional rupture of the peroneal tendon is often found, which may be associated with a prolonged varus deformity of the ankle; if it is found, all abnormal-appearing tendon should be debrided and tubularized.

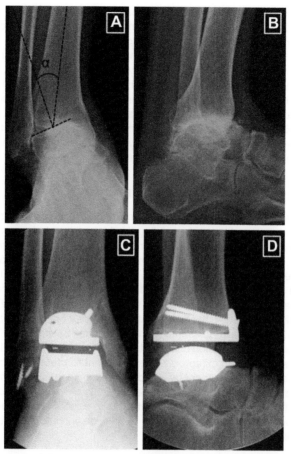

Fig. 2. Anteroposterior (*A*) and lateral (*B*) radiographs demonstrating a severe varus deformity (α = 30°). Anterioposterior (*C*) and lateral (*D*) radiographs after complete deformity correction with total ankle replacement (HINTEGRA Total Ankle Prosthesis, Newdeal, Lyon, France) combined with a modified Broström lateral ankle ligament plication procedure.

CALCANEAL OSTEOTOMY

After ligamentous imbalance has been managed, the alignment of the hindfoot should indicate whether to perform calcaneal osteotomy. Frequently, varus deformity of the hindfoot is associated with varus ankle osteoarthrosis. Correcting the hindfoot deformity before or simultaneously with total ankle replacement is essential for optimal long-term results. Numerous calcaneal osteotomies have been reported to demonstrate good clinical results, such as the lateral displacement osteotomy that translates the posterior fragment 5 to 10 mm laterally; the triplanar osteotomy[27] that corrects all 3 planes of cavovarus deformity by lateral translation of the tuberosity fragment coupled with lateral closing wedge osteotomy to correct the varus and proximal sliding of the tuberosity fragment to correct the calcaneal posture of the hindfoot and subtalar arthrodesis. The lateral closing wedge osteotomy was introduced by Dwyer.[28] It has commonly been used for the correction of the heel varus in combination with total ankle replacement, because it is technically easy and takes only a few extra minutes. To do so, a short, lateral, oblique incision is made directly posterior to the peroneus tendons, performing a lateral-based wedge osteotomy and tapering the wedge to, but not through, the medial cortex. After closing the gap, correction of the varus deformity is ensured. While holding the osteotomy in the desired position, insert 2 guide pins to determine the correct position for insertion of the cannulated cancellous screws. When the first pin engages the proximal fragment, a bone hook can help to pull the guide pin laterally to minimize the gap and to compress the bony surfaces together. Two 6.5-mm cancellous screws with partial thread are inserted perpendicular to the osteotomy site and started slightly posterior and lateral on the tuberosity segment, angled anteriorly and slightly medially.

DORSIFLEXION OSTEOTOMY OF THE FIRST METATARSAL

Once the ankle and hindfoot alignment is corrected, the surgeon should inspect the level of the metatarsal heads by holding the foot in a neutral position. Correction of hindfoot and ankle varus can drive plantarflexion of the first ray. As the plantarflexed first ray forces the heel and ankle into varus,[29] a dorsal closing wedge osteotomy should be done on the first metatarsal with total ankle replacement. Through a small incision on the dorsum of the first metatarsal base, approximately 1 cm distal to the first tarsal-metatarsal joint, a dorsal-based wedge of bone is removed with a sagittal saw. When making the cuts in the first metatarsal, angle it obliquely to allow for easier screw insertion. The most troublesome complication has been transfer metatarsalgia, attributable to excess dorsiflexion of the distal fragment, resulting from too much bone resection. Once creating an osteotomy, it is important to preserve enough of a proximal fragment for screw placement by avoiding beginning the osteotomy too close to the first tarsal-metatarsal joint. After the metatarsal is elevated, 2 guide pins can be inserted from the proximal-dorsal to plantar-distal aspect of the metatarsal. Two headless compression screws are inserted over guide wires to engage both cortices for maximal compression.

HEEL CORD LENGTHENING

Patients with end-stage ankle arthrosis who undergo total ankle replacement often have a contracture of the gastrocnemius-soleus complex. Recognition of tight heel cord is also possible by observing the limitation of ankle dorsiflexion with a trial component. If a minimal dorsiflexion of 10° cannot be achieved through total ankle replacement, heel cord lengthening can be considered. It can be achieved by either gastrocnemius recession or percutaneous tendo-Achilles tendon lengthening, depending on the results of the Silverskiöld test.

GASTROCNEMIUS RECESSION

Gastrocnemius recession, also known as the Strayer procedure, is a treatment option for patients who have heel cord tightness in which the chief cause of contracture is in the gastrocnemius alone. A posterior longitudinal incision is made over the middle of the calf at the level of the musculotendinous junction. After the aponeurosis of the gastrocnemius is exposed, a transverse incision is made through it. The surgeon can control tension by dorsiflexing the ankle to the desired angle (>10°). The paratenon and deep fascia are then carefully repaired to prevent adhesion to the overlying skin.

PERCUTANEOUS LENGTHENING OF THE ACHILLES TENDON

Tendo-Achilles tendon lengthening is indicated when both the gastrocnemius and soleus contribute to heel cord tightness through an open or percutaneous approach. Percutaneous teno-Achilles tendon lengthening is usually performed by the triple hemisection technique, described in detail by Hatt and Lamphier.[30] We prefer percutaneous tendo-Achilles lengthening rather than open procedures because this procedure is quick and free of complications,[31] and is easy to combine with total ankle replacement. Regardless of approach, care must be taken to avoid complete rupture of the Achilles tendon that can occur during overzealous dorsiflexion of the ankle.

HINDFOOT FUSION

Patients with end-stage arthrosis of the ankle joint frequently involve not only malalignment in the coronal plane, but also degenerative change or deformity affecting the adjacent joints.[15,16,19] For these reasons, total ankle replacement occasionally requires adjunctive procedures to the hindfoot along with aforementioned procedures to obtain a plantigrade foot. Poor results for total ankle replacement have been reported in younger and higher demand patients with hindfoot arthrodesis.[32] Performing various hindfoot fusions simultaneously with total ankle replacement or as a staged operation before total ankle replacement, Kim et al[17] recently reported good midterm outcome in their attempt to address the challenges of hindfoot arthritis and deformity in total ankle replacement.

Subtalar fusion and/or talonavicular fusion is most frequently combined with total ankle replacement.[17,33] If necessary, it can also be performed with triple arthrodesis to create a plantigrade foot in total ankle replacement. The calcaneocuboid joint is usually spared if there is no evidence of arthrosis, because sparing of this joint can reduce nonunion[34,35] and further adjacent joint arthritis.[36,37]

Hindfoot procedures can be performed as simultaneous or staged operations. However, arthrodesis of the hindfoot combined with total ankle replacement would be too extensive of a surgery for a patient's limb to tolerate in a single setting. Therefore, the patient's condition and the surgeon's skill should be considered when combining these procedures with total ankle replacement simultaneously.

CORRECTION OF VALGUS ANKLE DEFORMITY

Valgus ankle deformity is rare and often associated with malunion after ankle fractures and with posterior tibial tendon dysfunction. The most common scenario of malunion after ankle factures is a shortening and external rotation of the fibula, which can develop if fixation of the fibula is inadequate.[38] To correct valgus ankle deformity, a transverse osteotomy is made above the level of the syndesmosis through a lateral transmalleolar approach. The syndesmosis then should be opened and pulled down using a bone reduction clamp to distract the lateral malleolus distally. Autologous iliac crest bone graft or structural allograft bone graft is interposed into the osteotomy site, whereas the distal segment is distracted. It is fixed using plate and screws. It can be difficult to determine the required amount of lengthening and the rotational correction of the fibula (**Fig. 3**). Comparison with the radiographs of the contralateral ankle or the articular contact between the fibula and the lateral edge of the talus can help to judge the appropriate amount of correction.

Most valgus deformities are secondary to advanced posterior tibial tendon dysfunction. The progressive deformity results in forefoot supination with medial column instability and eventually pes planovalgus. The foot deformity must be managed

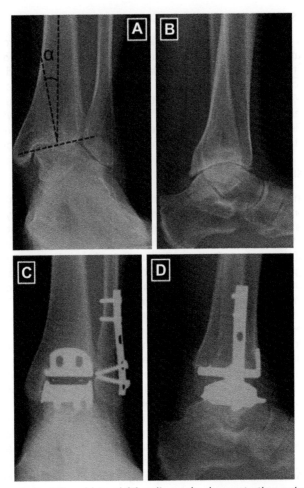

Fig. 3. Anteroposterior (*A*) and lateral (*B*) radiographs demonstrating a significant valgus deformity ($\alpha = 11°$) along with shortening of the fibula owing to malunion. Anteroposterior (*C*) and lateral (*D*) radiographs after complete deformity correction with total ankle replacement (HINTEGRA Total Ankle Prosthesis, Newdeal, Lyon, France) combined with lengthening osteotomy of the fibula.

before addressing the ankle to obtain a stable plantigrade foot. The procedures to correct posterior tibial tendon dysfunction include medial displacement calcaneal osteotomy, lateral column lengthening, soft-tissue procedures (eg, flexor digitorum longus tendon transfer, repair of the deltoid and spring ligament) and/or plantarflexion osteotomy of the first ray. In patients with rigid fixed deformity of the hindfoot, multiple arthrodeses are considered the procedures of choice, including isolated subtalar arthrodesis, isolated talonavicular arthrodesis, talonavicular and calcaneocuboid arthrodesis, and triple arthrodesis.[39] These procedures can shift the heel contact point laterally to obtain a plantigrade, stable foot, reducing stress on the lateral tibiotalar joint. The algorithm that is suggested for the treatment of a valgus ankle is shown in **Fig. 4.**

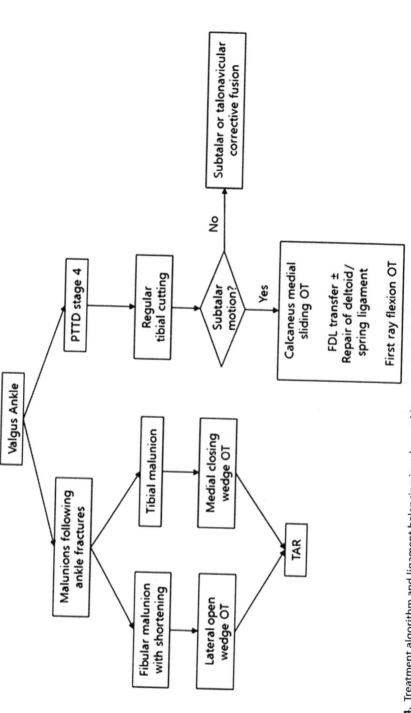

Fig. 4. Treatment algorithm and ligament balancing in valgus ankle osteoarthritis. Malunion after ankle fractures requires corrective osteotomy. Posterior tibial tendon dysfunction leading to a valgus ankle deformity. Total ankle replacement must be followed by additional correction of posterior tibial tendon dysfunction deformity.

POSTOPERATIVE CARE AND REHABILITATION

Patients are placed in a well-padded, short leg splint for 2 weeks. Suction drains can usually be removed the day after the operation, and sutures can be removed at postoperative day 14. In patients with uncomplicated total ankle replacement, a short leg cast is applied for 4 weeks. If additional procedures were performed, a short leg cast should be applied for a maximum of 6 weeks. At that time, the cast can be removed and the first postoperative radiographs taken. If a stable implant position and satisfactory healing of additional procedures are seen, the patient should be advised to increase weight-bearing as tolerated and gradually return to preoperative activities. Rehabilitation programs should be undertaken with exercises to improve muscular strength and muscular control of ankle movements.

CLINICAL RESULTS IN THE LITERATURE

There are several reports of successful total ankle replacement for varus or valgus unstable arthritic ankles in the literature. Although technically more demanding because of the need to perform additional procedures, total ankle replacement with coronal deformity of ankle, with short- to mid-term follow-up, demonstrates near-equal success with that of ankles with neutral alignment. Surgeons should use these studies as a guide regarding the success of the techniques discussed herein.

Doets et al[40] performed 15 primary total ankle replacements along with medial malleolar lengthening osteotomy to correct varus deformity in mainly rheumatoid arthritic ankles. Overall, outcomes were satisfactory in 86% of ankles after a mean follow-up of 5 years, and only 2 cases of osteotomy nonunion and 2 cases of gutter impingement requiring debridement were reported as complications. Hobson et al[12] treated 123 ankles with total ankle replacement, comparing 2 different groups: (1) Patients with preoperative coronal deformity greater than 10° and (2) patients with less than 10° of deformity. They evaluated the patients at a mean follow-up of 4 years and reported no difference between the 2 groups regarding postoperative range of motion, complications, or failure rates. The authors concluded that adequate correction of alignment and instability is important to achieving satisfactory clinical results in patients with a hindfoot deformity of up to 30°. Kim et al[13] also retrospectively reviewed the outcomes of surgery on 23 ankles with varus deformity of greater than or equal to 10° in comparison with 22 neutral ankles. The authors performed various additional procedures simultaneously with total ankle replacement to correct any accompanying malalignment, joint contracture, or instability. After a mean follow-up of 27 months, there were no differences between the 2 groups regarding clinical and radiologic outcomes. They concluded that satisfactory clinical outcomes can be achieved in varus ankles when performing total ankle replacement if effort is given to correct accompanying deformities.

SUMMARY

Ligament balancing in total ankle replacement is a vital portion of the operative procedure, and its effectiveness directly influences the quality of the replacement. Recent work on balancing of varus and valgus ankles has supported the notion of additional procedures based on function and range of motion of the ankle. Thus, for patients with varus or valgus deformed ankles, additional procedures should be performed to reconstruct to a neutral ankle joint. Surgeons should have the option to correct deformities of the ankle at the time of index surgical intervention. We believe that surgeons can achieve good alignment and optimal soft-tissue balance in ankles with moderate to severe varus or valgus alignment by using the above mentioned algorithms, which include various additional procedures combined with total ankle replacement.

REFERENCES

1. Buechel FF Sr, Buechel FF Jr, Pappas MJ. Ten-year evaluation of cementless Buechel-Pappas meniscal bearing total ankle replacement. Foot Ankle Int 2003;24(6):462–72.
2. Buechel FF Sr, Buechel FF Jr, Pappas MJ. Twenty-year evaluation of cementless mobile-bearing total ankle replacements. Clin Orthop Relat Res 2004;424:19–26.
3. Kofoed H. Scandinavian total ankle replacement (STAR). Clin Orthop Relat Res 2004;424:73–9.
4. Hintermann B, Valderrabano V, Dereymaeker G, et al. The HINTEGRA ankle: rationale and short-term results of 122 consecutive ankles. Clin Orthop Relat Res 2004;424:57–68.
5. Hintermann B, Valderrabano V, Knupp M, et al. The HINTEGRA ankle: short- and mid-term results. Orthopade 2006;35(5):533–45 [in German].
6. Doets HC, Brand R, Nelissen RG. Total ankle arthroplasty in inflammatory joint disease with use of two mobile-bearing designs. J Bone Joint Surg Am 2006; 88(6):1272–84.
7. Haskell A, Mann RA. Ankle arthroplasty with preoperative coronal plane deformity: short-term results. Clin Orthop Relat Res 2004;424:98–103.
8. Wood PL, Deakin S. Total ankle replacement. The results in 200 ankles. J Bone Joint Surg Br 2003;85(3):334–41.
9. Wood PL, Prem H, Sutton C. Total ankle replacement: medium-term results in 200 Scandinavian total ankle replacements. J Bone Joint Surg Br 2008;90(5):605–9.
10. Wood PL, Sutton C, Mishra V, et al. A randomised, controlled trial of two mobile-bearing total ankle replacements. J Bone Joint Surg Br 2009;91(1):69–74.
11. Takakura Y, Tanaka Y, Kumai T, et al. Ankle arthroplasty using three generations of metal and ceramic prostheses. Clin Orthop Relat Res 2004;424:130–6.
12. Hobson SA, Karantana A, Dhar S. Total ankle replacement in patients with significant pre-operative deformity of the hindfoot. J Bone Joint Surg Br 2009;91(4): 481–6.
13. Kim BS, Choi WJ, Kim YS, et al. Total ankle replacement in moderate to severe varus deformity of the ankle. J Bone Joint Surg Br 2009;91(9):1183–90.
14. Kim BS, Lee JW. Total ankle replacement for the varus unstable osteoarthritic ankle. Tech Foot Ankle Surg 2010;9(4):157.
15. Conti SF, Wong YS. Complications of total ankle replacement. Clin Orthop Relat Res 2001;(391):105–14.
16. Gould JS, Alvine FG, Mann RA, et al. Total ankle replacement: a surgical discussion. Part I. Replacement systems, indications, and contraindications. Am J Orthop 2000;29(8):604–9.
17. Kim BS, Knupp M, Zwicky L, et al. Total ankle replacement in association with hindfoot fusion: outcome and complications. J Bone Joint Surg Br 2010;92(11): 1540–7.
18. Espinosa N, Walti M, Favre P, et al. Misalignment of total ankle components can induce high joint contact pressures. J Bone Joint Surg Am 2010;92(5):1179–87.
19. Hintermann B. Total ankle arthroplasty: historical overview, current concepts, and future perspectives. New York: Springer; 2005.
20. Myerson MS. Reconstructive foot and ankle surgery: management of complications. St Louis (MO): Saunders/Elsevier; 2010.

21. Larsen A, Dale K, Eek M. Radiographic evaluation of rheumatoid arthritis and related conditions by standard reference films. Acta Radiol 1977;18(4):481–91.
22. Bonasia DE, Dettoni F, Femino JE, et al. Total ankle replacement: why, when and how? Iowa Orthop J 2010;30:119–30.
23. Clare MP, Sanders RW. Preoperative considerations in ankle replacement surgery. Foot Ankle Clin 2002;7(4):709–20.
24. Choi WJ, Lee JW. Heterotopic ossification after total ankle arthroplasty. J Bone Joint Surg Br 2011;93(11):1508–12.
25. Broström L. Sprained ankles. VI. Surgical treatment of "chronic" ligament ruptures. Acta Chir Scand 1966;132(5):551–65.
26. Kilger R, Knupp M, Hintermann B. Peroneus longus to peroneus brevis tendon transfer. Tech Foot Ankle Surg 2009;8(3):146.
27. Myerson M. Current therapy in foot and ankle surgery. St Louis (MO): B.C. Decker; 1993.
28. Dwyer FC. Osteotomy of the calcaneum for pes cavus. J Bone Joint Surg Br 1959;41(1):80–6.
29. Paulos L, Coleman SS, Samuelson KM. Pes cavovarus. Review of a surgical approach using selective soft-tissue procedures. J Bone Joint Surg Am 1980; 62(6):942–53.
30. Hatt RN, Lamphier TA. Triple hemisection: a simplified procedure for lengthening the Achilles tendon. N Engl J Med 1947;236(5):166–9.
31. Moreau MJ, Lake DM. Outpatient percutaneous heel cord lengthening in children. J Pediatr Orthop 1987;7(3):253–5.
32. Valderrabano V, Hintermann B, Dick W. Scandinavian total ankle replacement: a 3.7-year average followup of 65 patients. Clin Orthop Relat Res 2004;424:47–56.
33. Rippstein PF, Huber M, Coetzee JC, et al. Total ankle replacement with use of a new three-component implant. J Bone Joint Surg Am 2011;93(15):1426–35.
34. Graves SC, Mann RA, Graves KO. Triple arthrodesis in older adults. Results after long-term follow-up. J Bone Joint Surg Am 1993;75(3):355–62.
35. Sammarco VJ, Magur EG, Sammarco GJ, et al. Arthrodesis of the subtalar and talonavicular joints for correction of symptomatic hindfoot malalignment. Foot Ankle Int 2006;27(9):661–6.
36. Astion DJ, Deland JT, Otis JC, et al. Motion of the hindfoot after simulated arthrodesis. J Bone Joint Surg Am 1997;79(2):241–6.
37. Knupp M, Schuh R, Stufkens SA, et al. Subtalar and talonavicular arthrodesis through a single medial approach for the correction of severe planovalgus deformity. J Bone Joint Surg Br 2009;91(5):612–5.
38. Perera A, Myerson M. Surgical techniques for the reconstruction of malunited ankle fractures. Foot Ankle Clin 2008;13(4):737–51.
39. Myerson MS. Adult acquired flatfoot deformity: treatment of dysfunction of the posterior tibial tendon. Instr Course Lect 1997;46:393–405.
40. Doets HC, van der Plaat LW, Klein JP. Medial malleolar osteotomy for the correction of varus deformity during total ankle arthroplasty: results in 15 ankles. Foot Ankle Int 2008;29(2):171–7.

The INBONE II Total Ankle System

Bradley P. Abicht, DPM, Thomas S. Roukis, DPM, PhD*

KEYWORDS

- Arthroplasty • INBONE • Joint pain • Joint replacement • Tibiotalar joint

KEY POINTS

- Advancements in implant design, surgeon experience, and patient selection have led to improved outcomes in total ankle replacement, making it a viable alternative to ankle arthrodesis.
- Apart from being only 1 of 4 Food and Drug Administration (FDA)-approved ankle implants in the United States, the INBONE II Total Ankle System boasts a unique tibial intramedullary modular stem fixation structure characterized by customizable length patterns specific to patient anatomy and a talar component with sulcus articulating geometry that provides increased coronal plane stability.
- Preoperative templating gives surgeons an estimate of the size and position of the desired implant, but the final position and size should be determined intraoperatively through direct visualization and confirmed with multiple views using image intensification.
- Proper alignment with anterior-posterior and medial-lateral guide rods is pivotal for the success of the remaining steps of the case.
- Gentle tissue handling and proper execution of step-by-step technique lead to fewer complications, better outcomes, and increased survivorship of the implant.
- Adherence to a strict postoperative protocol is imperative to achieve optimal outcomes for both patients and surgeons, with ongoing periodic surveillance to check for any untoward signs of complication or impending failure.
- Despite significant improvements in total ankle replacement, patients should be well informed preoperatively of the potential for complications, including the risks versus benefits of proceeding with total ankle replacement.

INTRODUCTION

Total ankle replacement has witnessed resurgence in popularity over the past decade, making it a viable alternative to ankle arthrodesis and other definitive surgical treatments for debilitating tibiotalar joint pathology. Third-generation implants demonstrate advances in implant design, are less constrained, and rely on noncemented fixation for

Department of Orthopaedics, Podiatry, and Sports Medicine, Gundersen Lutheran Healthcare System, 2nd Floor Founders Building, 1900 South Avenue, La Crosse, WI 54601, USA
* Corresponding author. Department of Orthopaedics, Podiatry, and Sports Medicine, Gundersen Lutheran Healthcare System, 2nd Floor Founders Building, 1900 South Avenue, Mail Slot FB2-009, La Crosse, WI 54601.
E-mail address: tsroukis@gundluth.org

Clin Podiatr Med Surg 30 (2013) 47–68
http://dx.doi.org/10.1016/j.cpm.2012.08.006
0891-8422/13/$ – see front matter © 2013 Elsevier Inc. All rights reserved.

increased stability. These advances, in combination with improved surgeon training, a less formidable learning curve, better surgical instrumentation guiding implantation, and more clearly defined patient selection, have translated to lower implant failure rates with improved outcomes for primary and revision total ankle replacement cases. Furthermore, a recent literature review of implant survivorship reports ranges from 70% to 98% at 3 to 6 years and from 80% to 95% at 8 to 12 years.[1]

One implant, responsible in part for the aforementioned advancements, is the INBONE Total Ankle system (Wright Medical Technology, Arlington, Tennessee), more specifically, the company's current model, the INBONE II Total Ankle System. This implant remains 1 of 4 designs in the United States cleared by the FDA and in widespread clinical use. The INBONE (http://documents.wmt.com/Document/Get/FA180-308; accessed July 1, 2012) and INBONE II (http://documents.wmt.com/Document/Get/FA093-210; accessed July 1, 2012) total ankle systems are based on previous success achieved in other total joints, mainly the knee, and boast a unique intramedullary tibial stem composed in modular fashion and introduced into the distal tibial metaphysis (http://www.inbone.com/DesignRationale.aspx; accessed July 1, 2012).[2] The INBONE total ankle replacement, formally marketed as the Topez Total Ankle Replacement, became FDA 510(k) cleared in November 2005 (http://www.fda.gov/MedicalDevices/ProductsandMedicalProcedures/DeviceApprovalsandClearances/510kClearances/ucm089876.htm?utm_campaign=Google2&utm_source=fdaSearch&utm_medium=Web site&utm_term=topez%20total%20ankle%20replacement&utm_content=6; accessed July 1, 2012) and the INBONE II Total Ankle System became FDA 510(k) cleared in August 2010 (http://www.fda.gov/MedicalDevices/ProductsandMedicalProcedures/DeviceApprovalsandClearances/510kClearances/ucm239168.htm?utm_campaign=Google2&utm_source=fdaSearch&utm_medium=Web site&utm_term=inbone%20II%20total%20ankle%20replacement&utm_content=4; accessed July 1, 2012). Interconnecting stem pieces allow surgeons to build a tibial stem to custom length, which provides optimal strength and stability by dispersing bone implant interface. For the INBONE Total Ankle System, two anterior-posterior lengths exist for each size tibial tray to allow improved fit and coverage of anterior and posterior tibial cortices without the need for further bone resection from the medial or lateral malleoli. Also, for the INBONE II Total Ankle System, the talar component boasts a sulcus design to its proximal articulating aspect and a central stem with 2 4-mm anterior talar dome pegs to its distal surface. The sulcus articulating geometry provides increased coronal plane stability, permitting liberal medial and lateral gutter débridement (http://www.wmt.com/footandankle/FA701-1210.asp; accessed July 1, 2012).[3] The talar component's central stem and anterior pegs provide 3 points of fixation resulting in increased rotational stability (http://www.wmt.com/footandankle/FA701-1210.asp; accessed July 1, 2012). Four ultra–high-molecular-weight polyethylene (UHMWPE) insert thicknesses are available for each size implant, including two standard and two thicker revision UHMWPE inserts, which is particularly advantageous in the setting of total ankle replacement revision. A greater thickness of the polyethylene insert in combination with a broader constrained design of the INBONE II Total Ankle System results in less edge-loading effect and reduced delamination wear of the UHMWPE insert. The implant is FDA indicated for use with polymethylmethacrylate cement.

Despite significant design improvements established by the INBONE II Total Ankle system, indications and contraindications for total ankle replacement must be considered no matter which implant is preferred. Degenerative, inflammatory, and posttraumatic arthritis of the ankle remain the primary indications for total ankle replacement. Various investigators have noted that the results of total ankle replacement may be less favorable in patients with posttraumatic arthritis versus patients with either primary osteoarthritis or inflammatory arthritis.[4–6] In addition to arthritis as a cause, age is a relative contraindication, with total ankle replacement ideally involving patients 55 years or older. In a study involving 303 total ankle replacements, investigators reported implant survivorship of 74% and 89% for patients under and over, respectively, age 54 years.[7] Furthermore, patients with a median age of 54 or less had a 1.45-times greater risk for reoperation and a 2.65-times greater risk of implant failure than patients over age 54.[7] Preoperative deformity and/or ankle instability must also be assessed. In various studies involving mobile bearing implants, investigators noted that as coronal plane deformity increases, the survivorship of the implant generally decreases.[8,9] Adjunctive procedures, such as hindfoot or midfoot arthrodesis, lateral ankle stabilization, calcaneal osteotomy, or forefoot procedures, may be required to balance the foot and create a stable plantigrade pedal structure. Further contraindications of total ankle replacement include active infection, severe peripheral vascular disease, unresectable osteonecrotic bone, Charcot joints, and peripheral neuropathy.[10] As with any operative procedure, it is imperative that surgeons consider the aforementioned indications/contraindications and further adjunctive procedures that may be required on a patient-specific basis, because these factors greatly influence patient final outcome.

SURGICAL TECHNIQUE
Preoperative Planning

Once a patient has been determined a good candidate for primary or revision total ankle replacement with the INBONE II Total Ankle system, standard weight-bearing radiographs of the symptomatic foot and ankle are obtained. These include anterior-posterior, oblique, and lateral views of the foot as well as anterior-posterior, mortise, and lateral views of the ankle. Additionally, a hindfoot alignment view can be helpful when determining the rearfoot to leg relationship. Anterior-posterior and lateral long leg views of the leg encompassing the entire tibia and fibula may be beneficial in settings of previous trauma or revision surgery. Advanced imaging is sometimes used on a case-by-case basis. CT scans can help determine the extent of cystic changes and characterize the quality of cortical and cancellous bone structure, emphasizing areas of bone loss and deformity. It also benefits surgeons by illustrating the extent of concomitant arthritis within the subtalar or midfoot joints when determining adjunctive procedure selection. MRI may be beneficial to assess for the presence of active infection or widespread talar osteonecrosis, which are both contraindications to total ankle replacement.[10] Additionally, it may divulge information regarding the integrity of soft tissue structures functioning around the ankle.

Preoperative templating gives surgeons an estimate of the appropriate size and position of the tibial and talar components. The INBONE II Total Ankle System offers radiographic overlays, available in 0% and 10% magnifications, which represent both the anterior-posterior and lateral profiles of the prosthesis. This templating process should be used for estimation purposes only, because final component size and position should be determined intraoperatively using direct visualization and confirmed with intraoperative image intensification.

Prep and Patient Positioning

In the preoperative holding area, a regional local anesthetic block is performed by the anesthesia care team provider in the form of popliteal sciatic nerve block. An additional infiltration of local anesthetic to the region of the saphenous nerve distribution at the same time is beneficial. The popliteal block is usually well tolerated by patients and considered an excellent adjunct in the multimodal approach to pain control, because it minimizes the need for intraoperative and postoperative reliance on narcotic pain medication.

Apart from the regional block, total ankle replacement procedures are typically accomplished under general anesthesia for safety purposes. Thus, once patients are intubated and their airway secured, they are placed on the operating room table in the supine position with the heels at the end of bed. An indwelling Foley catheter is placed and retained postoperatively until patients are removed from bed rest protocol. A well-padded and appropriately sized nonsterile pneumatic thigh tourniquet is applied to the proximal thigh of the ipsilateral operative ankle, although it is the authors' preference to avoid tourniquet use unless completely necessary and is routinely circumvented. A large gel bump can be placed under the ipsilateral hip to internally rotate the operative lower extremity, bringing the foot and ankle into neutral position with the toes pointed toward the ceiling. The contralateral lower extremity is well padded across its bony prominences, and it is secured down with bath blankets and taped with care to make sufficient room for the foot holder.

During patient intubation and positioning, it is helpful to have a member of the surgical team scrub in and assemble the foot and leg holder. This permits adequate time to confirm proper configuration of the guide rods, drill, and alignment system before skin incision. Image intensification in the form of a large fluoroscopic C-arm is positioned and draped for facilitation from the ipsilateral side of the operative lower extremity. The operative lower extremity is prepped in normal aseptic fashion from toes to midthigh, allowing access to the ipsilateral knee as a reference point. Prophylactic antibiosis, determined by patient drug allergies and regional susceptibility levels, is infiltrated before skin incision and inflation of tourniquet if one is used. An antibacterial impervious incise barrier is secured over the toes and forefoot.

Surgical Approach

Soft tissue dissection is accomplished without the patient ankle secured in the foot holder to facilitate access and create adequate exposure. Delicate soft tissue handling is essential throughout the duration of the case to reduce the potential for inducing wound-healing complications. Using a combination of blunt and sharp large self-retaining retractors placed specifically only on the deep tissues and not on the skin and promptly removed when not necessary have proved helpful in limiting further iatrogenic trauma to the skin margins. A standard utility anterior ankle incision approach is used. A linear incision extending approximately 125 mm is used with placement directly medial to the extensor hallucis longus tendon. It is imperative to avoid placement of this incision directly over the tibialis anterior or extensor hallucis tendons, because there is a high potential for developing wound-healing complications postoperatively if spasticity, or bowstringing, of these tendons is present. Superficially, the superficial peroneal nerve or its communicating branches should be identified and protected if permissible. Due to anatomic variants, the course of this nerve occasionally requires it to be sacrificed if it precludes adequate exposure and access to the ankle joint. This remains a point that patients should be informed of preoperatively and may result in an area of anesthesia or dysesthesia postoperatively about the dorsal medial forefoot. The extensor sheath is incised, but maintained, permitting repair at time of closure. The extensor retinaculum is incised longitudinally, carrying dissection deep within the interval of the extensor hallucis longus and tibialis anterior tendons. The anterior tibial tendon sheath is maintained. The anterior neurovascular bundle, including the dorsalis pedis artery and deep peroneal nerve, is protected and retracted laterally. A Cobb periosteal elevator can be introduced to facilitate subperiosteal dissection to fully expose the distal tibia, talus, and portion of the midfoot. Chronic synovitis, loose bodies, and anterior tibiotalar osteophytes are removed from the anterior ankle recess. Adequate visualization should include the distal tibia, medial and lateral malleoli, with extension into the ankle gutters and distally onto the talonavicular joint.

Intramedullary Alignment Guide

After proper assembly of the alignment gig has been confirmed and adequate exposure of the ankle joint achieved, the operative lower extremity is placed and secured within the foot holder (http://www.wmt.com/footandankle/FA214-408.asp; http://documents.wmt.com/Document/Get/FA180-308; accessed July 1, 2012). The plantar calcaneus should fully seat against the foot holder in a flat position. A gastrocnemius recession or percutaneous tendo-Achilles lengthening may be necessary to rest the heel flush against the foot holder confirming the foot is 90° relative to the leg. If the foot is left plantarflexed, this places the talus at risk for being cut posteriorly on a bias. The ankle is slightly oriented with 10° of internal rotation. This can be accomplished by placing a thin osteotome within the medial gutter and internally rotating the ankle until the osteotome is parallel to the side of the foot holder.[3,10,11] The authors prefer to place extra padding, in the form of sterile foam, plantar to the metatarsal heads and around the calf, to reduce pressure-induced deep tissue injury that can occur when the foot and leg are secured in the holder for extended periods of time. The calcaneus is temporarily fixed within the holder with 2 2.4-mm Steinmann pins. The forefoot blocks are adjusted and secured to maintain the internal rotation. Elastic stretch wrap is placed circumferentially to the forefoot and calf regions for stability. Achilles support is engaged as needed, and the intramedullary alignment rods are centered within the tibia through a lateral view (**Fig. 1**).

Next, the C-arm image intensifier is transitioned from an anterior-posterior position to obtain a mortise view of the ankle, and the alignment guide is placed parallel in the coronal plane with the intramedullary axis of the tibia. This ensures proper varus/valgus positioning. Subsequent movements involve medial-lateral translation referencing the anterior-posterior guide rods, aligning the guidance system centrally within the talus. Proper alignment may take extra time but is pivotal for the success of the

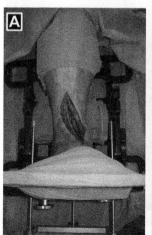
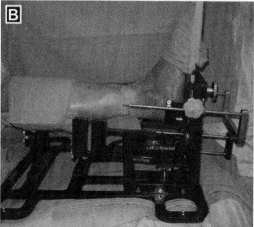

Fig. 1. Mortise (*A*) and lateral (*B*) views of the operative limb secured in the foot holder.

remaining steps of the case. Maneuvering between mortise and lateral views is often necessary and, if the leg holder, extremity, table, or C-arm image intensifier is moved inadvertently, the alignment can change. Thus, it is prudent to confirm proper alignment whenever doubt exists.

Once proper alignment is achieved (**Fig. 2**), the C-arm image intensifier is placed back to the mortise view. In various instances, ankle deformity may dictate the use of a lamina spreader strategically placed to properly align the talar plafond with the distal tibia.[3,10,11] The spreader is placed within the ankle joint in a medial position for varus deformities and lateral position for valgus deformity. This slightly distracts an arthritic joint and creates stability during the process of joint preparation. After confirmation of proper alignment with lateral and anterior-posterior views using anterior-posterior and medial-lateral guide rods, the process of joint resection and drilling can ensue.

Joint Resection

The drilling process ensues with placement of the primary bushing, collet, and cannula nut into the plantar foot holder. The tip of the trocar is inked with a surgical marker, and then the cannula with trocar is advanced through the primary bushing assembly to place an entry point marking onto the plantar foot. The cannula holder is then entirely removed, and through the hole in the foot holder a longitudinal linear incision extending approximately 2 cm is made just through skin. The surgeon should note that the incision placement is slightly medial to midline. A straight hemostat is inserted through soft tissues down to the calcaneus and then opened to clear a path for the subsequent cannula and drill. The primary bushing assembly is again threaded back into the foot

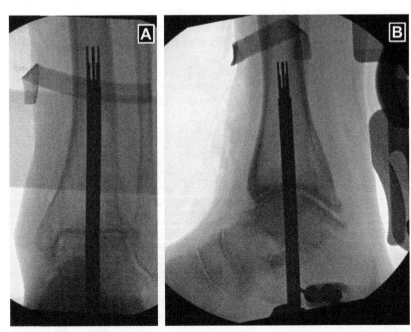

Fig. 2. Mortise (*A*) and lateral (*B*) image intensification C-arm images demonstrating proper alignment of the anterior-posterior (*A*) and lateral (*B*) alignment rods centered within the intramedullary axis of the tibia and talus.

holder, and the cannula with trocar is inserted and advanced with slight rotations back and forth until it abuts the calcaneus. The cannula is then locked in place with the cannula nut, and the trocar is removed. Anterior-posterior alignment is again verified while inserting a 6-mm drill bit through the cannula until it lightly abuts the calcaneus (**Fig. 3**). The drill is then started in reverse mode, and the surgeon peck drills through the calcaneus, talus, and tibia (**Fig. 4**). Once into the tibia, the drill can be advanced on forward while peck drilling. This process helps prevent skiving off the medial aspect of the calcaneus and creates a more accurate drill pattern. Serial mortise views obtained with C-arm image intensification while drilling should verify the drill follows the anterior-posterior centering guide, lying directly over it. Once into the tibia, continue the drill 5-cm to 7-cm proximal to the ankle joint or to the proper level as determined from preoperative templates depending on the number of stem pieces desired and patient anatomy. The drill and cannula are left in place, but the power drill driver is disconnected.

After the drilling process is complete, the anterior fixture with a properly sized saw cutting guide is mounted (**Fig. 5**). Using image intensification, the saw guide is centered over the drill, taking care not to compress the tissues of the anterior ankle. The proper size cut guide is one that aligns the medial arm of the cut guide with the medial gutter and spares the lateral malleolus in its entirety. Two saw blades are then manually placed, one into the proximal and one into the distal cut guide slots, and a lateral view is used to estimate that the proper amount of talus will be resected. If the guide requires more proximal repositioning, more of the malleoli is resected and the specific risk of medial malleolar fracture increases. Therefore, the medial-lateral alignment should be double-checked after any axial movement of the guide and the medial-lateral position corrected accordingly. Once alignment is confirmed, the saw guide is pinned to the tibia and talus, and blocking pins are placed to protect the malleoli (**Fig. 6**A, B). The previous mortise view can be used for proper insertion of the blocking pins and should be placed such that the lateral pin is between the talus and fibula and the medial pin is between the talus and medial malleolus. The peck drill is then withdrawn from the tibia but can be left within the calcaneus for stability. Next,

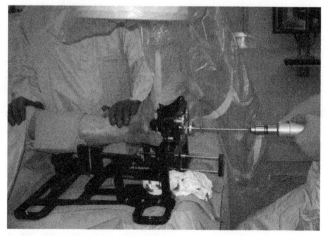

Fig. 3. Lateral view demonstrating drill inserted into the plantar calcaneus through the cannula secured to the foot holder. Note the additional support provided by the assistant and the use of image intensification C-arm images during drill advancement.

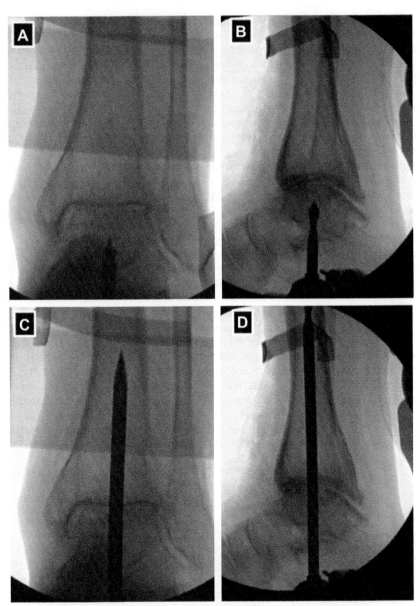

Fig. 4. Mortise (*A*) and lateral (*B*) image intensification C-arm images demonstrating entry of the drill into the talus. Mortise (*C*) and lateral (*D*) image intensification C-arm images demonstrating entry of the drill into the tibia to the level of intended reaming and stem insertion. Note that the anterior-posterior and lateral guide rods, respectively, would be used to verify correct trajectory of the drill throughout this process.

the antirotation block is placed in the cutting guide and the drill is used bicortical to pierce the anterior and posterior cortices of the tibia (see **Fig. 6**C, D). First the tibia is cut through the saw guide and then the talus. A lateral view can be used to check depth when pinning the tibia and talus or using the saw to complete the cuts. Finally,

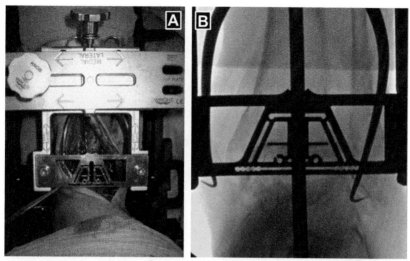

Fig. 5. Intraoperative anterior-posterior photograph (*A*) and image intensification C-arm mortise view (*B*) demonstrating the anterior fixture cutting guide that has been centered and secured to the foot holder.

the medial and lateral aspects of the tibia are then cut. It is imperative to have the saw blades parallel to the saw guide during all bone cuts.

Once the bone cuts are complete, the anterior cut guide is removed and the process of bone extraction proceeds. To start, an osteotome or saw can be used at the proximal tibial cut down toward the talus at an approximately 60° angle (**Fig. 7**A). Removing this anterior tibial section facilitates removal of the talar section in one piece by grabbing the retained Steinmann pins. The remaining Steinmann pins are pulled and retained bone removed. Several instruments are available to aid in bone removal, including a corner chisel, bone removal screw, and posterior capsule release tool. The corner chisel is helpful for saw passes that may not have been fully complete in the medial and/or lateral corners (see **Fig. 7**B, C). The bone removal screw can be inserted into larger fragments of bone and used as a joystick to toggle and manipulate the piece free (see **Fig. 7**D). The posterior capsule release tool can pass posterior to the remaining deep bone segments to help detach soft tissue attachments and is often the most difficult bone to remove in this process (see **Fig. 7**E, F) (http://documents. wmt.com/Document/Get/FA093-210; accessed July 1, 2012). The surgeon should take care not to lever medially or laterally when attempting bone removal, because the malleoli are at risk for fracture. A reciprocating saw and/or bone rasp should be used to fine-tune previous cuts to make completely flat surfaces. A drill can be used to redefine the antirotation notch as needed. Once all loose bone pieces have been removed and cut surfaces are flush, the joint should be copiously irrigated, which can be accomplished using pulse lavage irrigation system with or without antibiotic within the sterile saline solution (**Fig. 8**).

Implant Insertion

After successful bone extraction, the tibia can be reamed. The reamer tip is applied through the joint using power, placing it onto the tibial reamer drive rod, which is introduced through the calcaneus and talus. The surgeon must take care to avoid crossthreading the reamer tip. The tibia is then reamed by advancing the reamer tip,

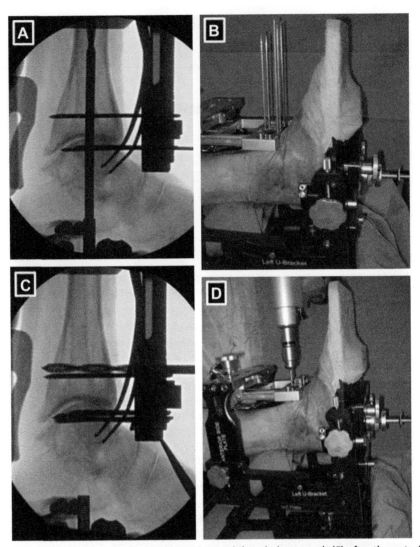

Fig. 6. Lateral image intensification C-arm image (*A*) and photograph (*B*) after the anterior fixture cutting guide has been pinned to the tibia and talus. Lateral image intensification C-arm image (*C*) and photograph (*D*) after the antirotation notch has been drilling bicortical through the anterior fixture cutting guide.

12-mm, 14-mm, or 16-mm in diameter, proximally to the appropriate level as determined preoperatively by the number of stem pieces that are used (**Fig. 9**). It is key to remember that the reamer should always be placed on forward (clockwise) when reaming proximally and also when extracting the reamer; otherwise, the reamer tip is at risk for disengaging and becoming lodged within the tibial canal. The joint should be copiously irrigated again after reaming is complete. The appropriate size tibial tray anterior-posterior trial sizer is selected and inserted into the resected joint space, and the strike rod may be used to fully seat the sizer into the resected tibia (**Fig. 10**).

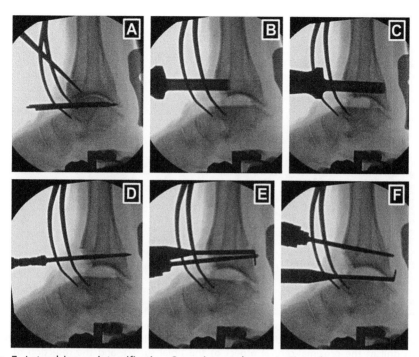

Fig. 7. Lateral image intensification C-arm image demonstrating placement of an osteotome from the transected distal tibia to the talus at an approximately 60° angle (A). This is followed by removal of the resected talar dome. The corner chisel is then placed into the medial corner (B) and gently tapped through the posterior aspect of the resected tibia under image intensification C-arm control (C). The bone removal screw is shown fully seated within the midsection of the transected distal tibia (D). This is followed by use of the posterior capsule release tool at the superior (E) and inferior (F) surfaces of the transected distal tibia to release remaining soft tissues.

A lateral view is checked for both standard and long sizing, ensuring that both the anterior and posterior cortices of the tibia are fully covered. This is most important anteriorly where most of the load is distributed. Once the appropriate tibial tray size is determined, the tibial stem is ready to be placed. The proximal conical stem piece and the first midstem piece can be assembled on the back table with an appropriately sized wrench and the x-drive screwdriver. At this point the surgeon should confirm the plantarflexion-dorsiflexion drill stop has been set for the footplate to return to the exact same position. The ankle is then plantarflexed to introduce the proximal tibial stem components, placing the nose of the conical piece within the tibial canal (**Fig. 11A**). The next midstem piece is introduced into the ankle joint with the clip, and the x-drive engages this piece to thread it to the first stem pieces (see **Fig. 11B**). The wrench is then moved to the most distal stem piece, and the stem is advanced proximally into the tibia. This process is repeated for additional midstem components (see **Fig. 11C**). The base stem piece is introduced similarly, but the surgeon must take care to rotate the morse taper release hole into an anterior-facing position, in line with the antirotation notch (see **Fig. 11D**). This release hole is used to detach the tibial base stem from the tibial tray in the event of revision. The wrench is left on the base stem, and the properly sized tibial tray is introduced with a holding tool inserting the

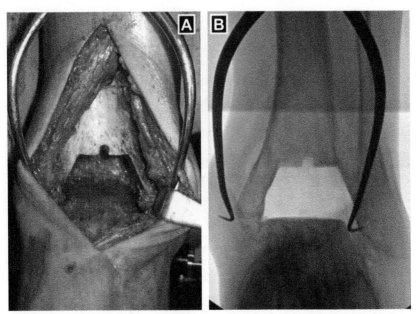

Fig. 8. Anterior-posterior photograph (*A*) and image intensification C-arm mortise view (*B*) after resection of the distal tibia and talus and copious irrigation. Note the antirotation notch drill at the proximal-central aspect of the tibial surface and the resection of the medial and lateral gutters to prevent impingement.

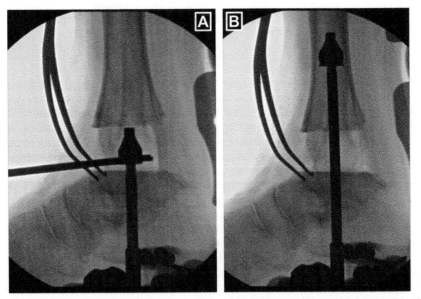

Fig. 9. Lateral image intensification C-arm view demonstrating the reamer tip held in the wrench and secured to the threaded rod (*A*) followed by proximal reaming to the level of intended stem insertion (*B*).

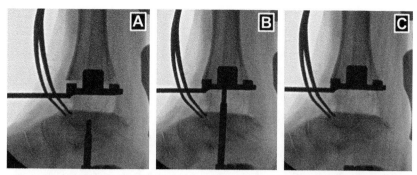

Fig. 10. Lateral image intensification C-arm view demonstrating initial insertion of the appropriate sized tibial tray sizer into the reamed section of the distal tibia and the anterior and posterior tabs centered within the antirotation drill hole (*A*). This is followed by seating the tibial tray sizer with the strike rod that has been introduced through the plantar foot (*B*). The anterior and posterior tibial cortices should be fully covered by the tibial tray and it should be fully seated against the distal tibia (*C*).

morse taper into the stem base. The strike rod is used against the distal surface of the tibial tray, and the holding tool is removed. The rod is struck with a mallet several times to seat the morse taper and then remove the wrench. Tobramycin-impregnated poly-methylmethacrylate bone cement is applied to the proximal and sidewall surfaces of the tibial tray component, avoiding placement to the anterior face or distal surface of the tray (**Fig. 12**A). The strike rod is used to push the tibial construct into the tibia and confirm proper alignment, sizing, and cortical bone coverage with both a lateral (see **Fig. 12**B) and mortise (see **Fig. 12**C) view using image intensification.

After proper installation of the tibial tray and tibial stem components, the talus can be reamed and sized accordingly. Depending on the tibial tray size, the surgeon has the option of the corresponding size for talar dome implant or one size smaller (**Fig. 13**). Both sizes of talar dome trials are inserted with the talar dome trial holding tool. Both mortise and lateral views are used to select the talar dome trial size that provides complete coverage from medial to lateral with minimal overhang as well as coverage from anterior to posterior cortical margins. The surgeon should ensure the medial and lateral gutters are sufficiently débrided and that no impingement exists. Once the appropriate size talar dome trial piece is determined, a trial UHMWPE insert is set into the tibial tray. The trial talar component is again placed over the residual talus so that complete coverage of the cortical rim is achieved with a congruent posterior slope maintained between the native talus and trial talar component as confirmed on lateral view with image intensification. The ankle is then placed through range of motion, and the talar component should settle into anatomic alignment. This should be confirmed with image intensification through a lateral and mortise view. Once the talar dome trial has settled into optimum anatomic position, it is secured with 2 1.4-mm pins for temporary fixation (**Fig. 14**A). The foot is then plantarflexed and the trial UHMWPE insert removed. The 4-mm anterior peg drill is then used to drill holes through the medial and lateral openings of the talar dome trial, and a hard stop design ensures proper drilling depth for the talar dome anterior pegs (see **Fig. 14**B). A 2.4-mm pin is then driven through the center of the talar dome trial to the depth of the selected talar stem that is either 10 mm or 14 mm and the depth is verified with a lateral image intensification view (see **Fig. 14**C). The 1.4-mm pins are then removed along with the talar dome trial, leaving the 2.4-mm, centrally placed pin. The appropriate length talar

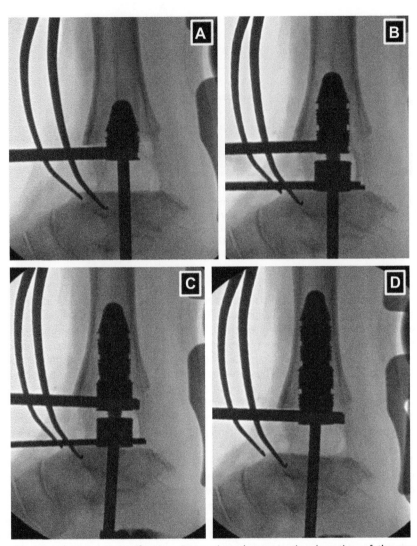

Fig. 11. Lateral image intensification C-arm view demonstrating insertion of the appropriate diameter stem top and midstem as 1 unit (*A*) followed by insertion of additional midstem components (*B, C*) and then the base stem (*D*).

stem reamer is then inserted over the 2.4-mm pin, and the talus is reamed to the depth of the selected talar stem (see **Fig. 14**D). A lateral view should be used to confirm depth, because the talar stem should not create subtalar joint impingement and it is not intended for subtalar joint arthrodesis fixation. As an option, the ENDO-FUSE Intraosseous Fusion System (Wright Medical Technology, Memphis, Tennessee) can be placed after preparing the subtalar joint for arthrodesis if desired but is not routine.[12,13] This may be ideal in cases with concomitant severe hindfoot arthrosis, when the talus is thin and osteoporotic, which provides fixation across the subtalar joint and aids in limiting subsidence of the talar component or in cases of revision total ankle replacement with subsidence of the talar component.[14] On the back table, the talar component is assembled on the strike block. The talar stem is then inserted into the talar dome,

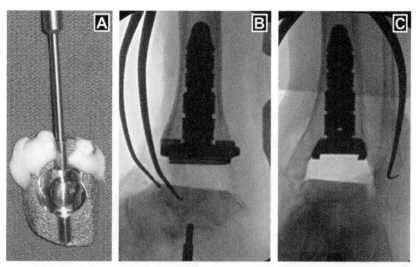

Fig. 12. Photograph demonstrating the superior surface of the tibial tray secured to the green insertion handle with Tobramycin-impregnated polymethylmethacrylate bone cement is applied to the proximal and sidewall surfaces (*A*). Lateral (*B*) and mortise (*C*) image intensification C-arm views after seating of the tibial tray into the base stem and impaction against the distal tibial resected surface.

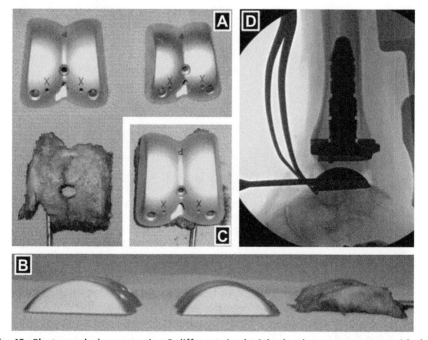

Fig. 13. Photograph demonstrating 2 different-sized trial talar dome components with the resected talus as seen from superior (*A*) and lateral (*B*) viewpoints. The larger of the 2 trial talar components is shown on-top of the resected talus with good coverage all around being evident (*C*). Lateral image intensification C-arm view with the trial talar dome component centered on top of the resected talus demonstrating good coverage (*D*).

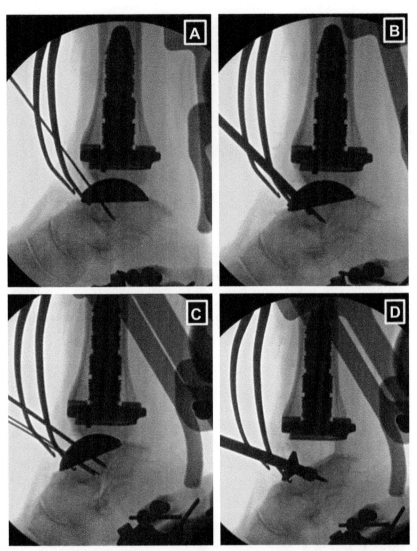

Fig. 14. Lateral image intensification C-arm view demonstrating proper placement of the talar component being secured with 2 1.4-mm pins (*A*) followed by 4-mm anterior peg drilling through the medial and lateral openings (*B*). Next, a 2.4-mm pin is driven through the center of the talar dome trial (*C*) that is left in place after removal of the remaining pins and talar trial component. The appropriate length talar stem reamer is then inserted and used to ream to the appropriate depth (*D*).

ensuring that the stem is parallel with the anterior pegs (**Fig. 15**A). Tobramycin-impregnated polymethylmethacrylate bone cement is again applied to the anterior portion of the distal surface of the talar component and anterior pegs (see **Fig. 15**B). The blue tray insert is placed within the tibial tray for protection. Using the talar holding tool, the talar component is inserted. The dome strike tool is used to fully seat the talar dome, and position is confirmed with mortise and lateral views. Any excess bone cement that is expressed should be removed. The foot holder is then removed from

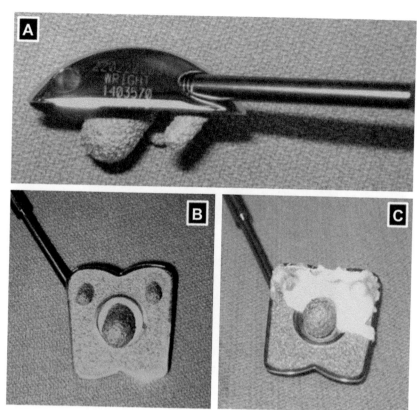

Fig. 15. Lateral photograph of the talar component secured to the purple insertion handle demonstrating the parallel alignment between the anterior pegs and stem (*A*). Photograph of the undersurface of the talar component is shown (*B*) followed by application of Tobramycin-impregnated polymethylmethacrylate bone cement to the anterior surfaces (*C*).

the operative lower extremity. The surgical site is copiously irrigated (as described previously). The appropriately sized trial UHMWPE insert is then placed securely into the joint space and articulation with the tibial tray is verified, followed by removal. The UHMWPE insertion tool is then assembled and used to insert the appropriately sized final insert (**Fig. 16**). In cases of coronal plane instability, a thicker UHMWPE insert should be used. Once the UHMWPE insertion tool bottoms out, it is removed and the UHMWPE is further seated with the UHMWPE impact tool striking it at a 60° angle. That the UHMWPE insert is fully seated is confirmed and range of motion is checked with dorsiflexion and plantarflexion of the ankle (**Fig. 17**). Inversion and eversion stability is also checked. Position of the implant and stability with range of motion and against anterior-posterior and inversion-eversion displacement can be confirmed through final mortise and lateral views using image intensification. Neutral, dorsiflexion, and plantar-flexion views of the ankle are saved to confirm range of motion (**Fig. 18**). The surgical site is copiously irrigated (as described previously) before final wound closure.

Closure

After pulse lavage irrigation, a closed suction surgical drain is sewn in place. The surgical wound is closed in layers, approximating the capsule and extensor

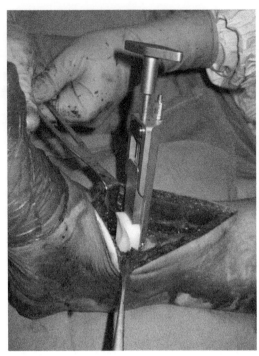

Fig. 16. Lateral photograph demonstrating the UHMWPE insert captured within the insertion tool.

retinaculum with 2–0 absorbable interrupted sutures. The subcutaneous layer is closed with buried 3–0 absorbable interrupted sutures. Skin margins are approximated under minimal tension with absorbable 3–0 nonabsorbable simple interrupted sutures or metallic skin staples. A well-padded sterile dressing is then applied from toes to knee with the addition of a plaster sugar tong and posterior slab dressing maintaining the foot at 90° to the lower leg or slight dorsiflexion of the ankle. Sterile foam is again incorporated into the postoperative surgical dressing, placing it over the anterior ankle incision, metatarsal head region, and any other bony prominence to avoid potential iatrogenic pressure necrosis. Specifics of the INBONE II Total Ankle System components implanted with proper sizes and lengths should be documented within the operative report for the tibial, talar, and UHMWPE insert for future reference.

POSTOPERATIVE PROTOCOL

Patients are admitted postoperatively and kept on strict bed rest protocol with lower extremities elevated above heart level and heels offloaded using pillow cocoon and bed positioning protocol, as described by Schweinberger and Roukis.[15] Supplemental oxygen via nasal cannula is helpful in reducing incision and ischemia-related wound-healing problems.[10] The suction drain is maintained until there is a less than 1-mm output per hour. A dressing change is then preformed where the splint is removed and incision site inspected for cardinal signs of infection, wound dehiscence, pressure necrosis, and other confounding factors. The surgical drain is removed. Patients are then placed into a well-padded short leg fiberglass cast with the foot at 90° to the leg, taking care to pad the same areas (as described previously). The indwelling Foley

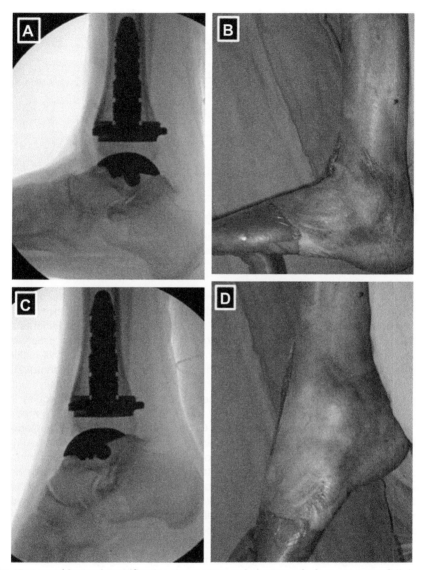

Fig. 17. Lateral image intensification C-arm view and photograph demonstrating full dorsi-flexion (*A, B*) and plantarflexion (*C, D*) range of motion, respectively.

catheter is removed if permissible, and patients are then permitted to initiate physical and occupational therapy, working on sit, stand, turn, and transfers to a bedside commode. Once patients can demonstrate competence with transfers and short-distance ambulation while maintaining strict non–weight bearing to the operative lower extremity, discharge to home versus a skilled nursing facility proceeds.

Patients maintain 100% strict non–weight bearing to the operative lower extremity for up to 8 weeks from the date of their surgical procedure to allow incision healing and osseous ongrowth to the implant components and continue with elevation above heart level to aid in edema control. They are instructed to continue to push incentive

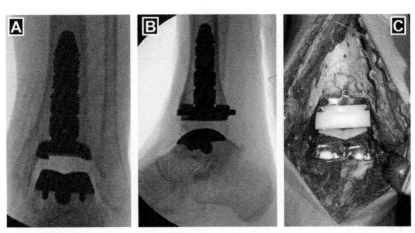

Fig. 18. Mortise (*A*) and lateral (*B*) image intensification C-arm views as well as anterior-posterior photograph (*C*) demonstrating final alignment before closure.

spirometry 10 times per hour when awake and perform upper extremity, core, and contralateral lower extremity exercises with resistance bands. This process starts postoperative day zero and continues until mobility is again achieved. Patients also continue on a strict mechanical and pharmacologic thromboembolic prophylaxis protocol until a return to full weight bearing and activity is realized. This includes continuing to don compressive thromboembolic deterrent hose to the contralateral lower extremity during waking hours of the day, aspirin (325-mg twice daily) (unless patients have a drug allergy or are deemed at higher risk and thus require low-molecular-weight heparin), getting up every hour during the day to maintain mobility, and staying well hydrated with clear fluids. Once anterior incision is fully healed and sutures are sequentially removed, patients are transitioned to a removable pneumatic airwalker fixed ankle long leg boot and permitted to remove it only for bathing purposes. At the 8-week follow-up appointment, the standard 3 views of the ankle in weight-bearing position are obtained to confirm alignment of the implant and ingrowth of surrounding bone. If no complications are noted with viable on-growth of implants, patients are permitted to transition into weight bearing on the operative lower extremity while using the removable boot. Once full weight bearing is achieved at 12 weeks, patients transition back to normal shoe gear, preferably a supportive tennis shoe or high-top boot. Weight-bearing follow-up radiographs with 3 standard views of the ankle are obtained with optional stress dorsiflexion and plantarflexion views at 1 year and every year thereafter.

COMPLICATIONS

Inherently, any surgery is at risk for complications, and total ankle replacement is no different. Improvements in surgical technique as well as better patient selection help reduce potential complications. Intraoperative complications are a possibility and include malleolar fractures, tibial, or talar fractures; iatrogenic tendon or neurovascular injuries; acute blood loss; iatrogenic pressure-induced necrosis; failure to recognize concomitant deformities; and thromboembolic events. Postoperatively, surgeons should be cognizant of wound-healing complications, infection potential, and continued pain and edema as well as the potential for thromboembolic events throughout the duration of immobilization. Patients are also placed on prophylactic oral antibiotic for life before routine dental cleanings or procedures. If an acute infection develops and is recognized early, irrigation and débridement with UHMWPE insert exchange is permitted in combination with prompt infectious disease consult. Chronic infections may require irrigation and débridement with explantation of components and placement of antibiotic spacer, with 6 weeks of intravenous antibiotic therapy followed by either revision total ankle replacement or conversion to ankle arthrodesis. Long-term complications may consist of component position changes, aseptic loosening, subsidence, ankle instability, impingement, UHMWPE insert wear, and the formation of cysts with osteolysis. Patients should be routinely followed for surveillance of developing complications, which can ultimately lead to implant failure or, less commonly, amputation of the leg.

SUMMARY

The INBONE II Total Ankle System is an FDA-approved total ankle implant that boasts a unique intramedullary alignment system with improved modular customizable tibial stem fixation. In addition, the sulcus articulating geometry of the talar component with broader polyethylene inserts imparts stability and creates a more even pressure gradient. These characteristics make this implant a desirable choice in both primary and revision cases. As with any surgery, patients should be well informed preoperatively of the potential for complications, including the risks versus benefits of proceeding with total ankle replacement.

REFERENCES

1. Easley ME, Adams SB, Hembree CW, et al. Results of total ankle arthroplasty. J Bone Joint Surg Am 2011;93:1455–68.
2. Reiley MA. INBONE total ankle replacement. Foot Ankle Spec 2008;1:118–22.
3. DeOrio JK. INBONE total ankle replacement: current status. Orthopaedic Knowledge Online: Foot and Ankle; 2011. Available at: http://orthoportal.org/oko/article.aspx?article=OKO_FOO036#abstract. Accessed July 1, 2012.
4. Bai LB, Lee KB, Song EK, et al. Total ankle arthroplasty outcome comparison for post-traumatic and primary osteoarthritis. Foot Ankle Int 2010;31:1048–56.
5. Naal FD, Impellizzeri FM, Loibl M, et al. Habitual physical activity and sports participation after total ankle arthroplasty. Am J Sports Med 2009;37:95–102.
6. Pyevich MT, Saltzman CL, Callaghan JJ, et al. Total ankle arthroplasty: a unique design. Two to twelve-year follow-up. J Bone Joint Surg Am 1998;80:1410–20.
7. Spirt AA, Assal M, Hansen ST Jr. Complications and failure after total ankle arthroplasty. J Bone Joint Surg Am 2004;86:1172–8.
8. Wood PL, Sutton C, Mishra V, et al. A randomized, controlled trial of two mobile-bearing total ankle replacements. J Bone Joint Surg Br 2009;91:69–74.
9. Doets HC, Brand R, Nelissen RG. Total ankle arthroplasty in inflammatory joint disease with use of two mobile-bearing designs. J Bone Joint Surg Am 2006;88:1272–84.
10. DeOrio JK. Focus on total ankle arthroplasty. Orthopedics 2006;29:978–80.
11. Ellis S, DeOrio JK. The INBONE total ankle replacement. Oper Tech Orthop 2010;20:201–10.
12. DeOrio JK. Total ankle replacement with subtalar arthrodesis. Management of combined ankle and subtalar arthritis. Tech Foot Ankle Surg 2010;9:182–9.

13. DeOrio JK. INBONE total ankle replacement: supplementary procedures. Orthopaedic Knowledge Online: Foot and Ankle; 2011. Available at: http://orthoportal.org/oko/article.aspx?article=OKO_FOO040#abstract. Accessed July 1, 2012.
14. Schuberth JM, Christensen JC, Rialson JA. Metal-reinforced cement augmentation for complex talar subsidence in failed total ankle arthroplasty. J Foot Ankle Surg 2011;50:766–72.
15. Schweinberger MH, Roukis TS. Effectiveness of instituting a specific bed protocol in reducing complications associated with bed rest. J Foot Ankle Surg 2010;49: 340–7.

Salto Talaris Fixed-Bearing Total Ankle Replacement System

Shannon M. Rush, DPM[a,b,*], Nicholas Todd, DPM[c]

KEYWORDS

- Arthroplasty • Salto • Joint pain • Joint replacement • Tibio-talar joint

KEY POINTS

- Apart from being only 1 of 4 Food and Drug Administration–approved ankle implants in the United States, the Salto Talaris total ankle system has moved the mobile-bearing concept from the implant to the instrumentation at the time of tibial trial.
- This was because of in situ motion analysis determination that very little movement (universally, <1 mm) occurred between the ultra-high molecular weight polyethylene insert and the tibial tray in the mobile-bearing Salto design used outside the United States.
- Additional design improvements include varying radii of the talar component to allow for physiologic tensioning of the medial and lateral collateral ligament complexes.
- Liberal use of image intensification, adherence to a perioperative protocol, and strict adherence to surgical technique, indications, and contraindications are essential for a quality outcome.

INTRODUCTION

Total ankle replacement has become a reliable and valuable procedure for patients who suffer from degenerative arthritis of the ankle joint. Historically, the only definitive option for treatment of end-stage degenerative arthritis was arthrodesis. Total ankle replacement has become a predictable alternative to arthrodesis that is credited to improving surgical technique, understanding surgical biomechanics of total ankle replacement, improved prosthesis design, and precision instrumentation.[1] Furthermore, total ankle replacement seems to have a preserving affect on the subtalar joint that are subject to further degenerative changes after ankle arthrodesis.[1–3] In addition, it seems that ankle arthrodesis leads to less favorable functional results and diminishing patient satisfaction.

[a] Silicon Valley Foot and Ankle Fellowship, Department of Podiatric Surgery, Palo Alto Medical Foundation, Mountain View, CA, USA; [b] Department of Podiatric Surgery, El Camino Hospital, Mountain View, CA, USA; [c] Department of Podiatric Surgery, Palo Alto Medical Foundation, Mountain View, CA, USA
* Corresponding author. Silicon Valley Foot and Ankle Fellowship, Department of Podiatric Surgery, Palo Alto Medical Foundation, Mountain View, CA.
E-mail address: Rushs1@PAMF.org

Clin Podiatr Med Surg 30 (2013) 69–80
http://dx.doi.org/10.1016/j.cpm.2012.09.002   **podiatric.theclinics.com**
0891-8422/13/$ – see front matter © 2013 Published by Elsevier Inc.

The Salto total ankle prothesis was designed in 1994 and was first used clinically in Europe in 1997.[4] The name Salto is derived from the Italian word for "jump." The design rationale was to construct a meniscal-bearing, cementless implant. The initial Salto prosthesis had remarkable clinical success.[5] It was further studied and revised after numerous cadaveric and retrospective evaluations.

SALTO TALARIS DESIGN

The Salto Talaris (Talaris is derived from the Italian word for "sandal") prosthesis received clearance for use with polymethylmethacrylate cement fixation in the United States by the Food and Drug Administration in 2006 (see http://www.accessdata.fda.gov/cdrh_docs/pdf9/K090076.pdf) (**Fig. 1**). The design was based on the initial successful experiences of the Salto mobile-bearing total ankle prosthesis in Europe. The mobile-bearing prosthesis showed 93% survivorship at a mean of 6.4 years.[5] Results of the Salto total ankle prosthesis were promising, yet designers decided to develop a fixed-bearing ankle prosthesis. The decision for transition to a fixed-bearing prosthesis was based on clinical and radiographic evaluation of 20 patients who received total ankle replacement. The mobile-bearing prosthesis experience showed that there was very little motion between the tibial component and the mobile-bearing ultra-high molecular weight polyethylene (UHMWPE) insert (Amy Ables, PhD, personal communication, July 2, 2012). Seventeen of the patients showed no anterior-to-posterior motion between the inferior surface of the tibial component and the superior surface of the UHMWPE insert. In the remaining 3 patients, there was less than 1 mm of motion. This demonstration essentially showed that the UHMWPE insert was not functioning as a mobile-bearing 3-component system and instead remained essentially fixed to the tibial prosthesis like a 2-component fixed-bearing system.[4]

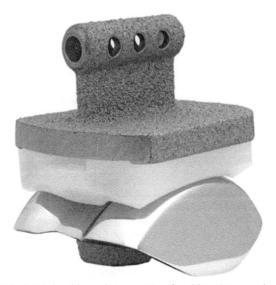

Fig. 1. The Salto Talaris total ankle replacement is a fixed-bearing prosthesis with anatomic design features. The talar component has varying radii of curvature that simulate the mechanical frustrum of the ankle with motion. The plasma titanium spray on the surface promotes ingrowth of bone and stable biologic fixation. The keel increases osseous contact.

Three-dimensional studies on 50 cadaveric studies helped redesign the tibial and talar components. The talar component was redesigned to a conical surface, with 2 radii of curvature. The differing radii allowed for equal tensioning of the collateral ligaments that provides mechanical stability for the prosthesis (**Fig. 2**). This is a critical adaptation for an anatomic designed prosthesis. There is often asymmetric laxity within the medial and lateral collateral ligament complexes. The varying radii of the talar component allow for physiologic tensioning throughout the total ankle range of motion. The redesigned talar component is designed with a sagittal groove, which directs transverse plane motion with dorsiflexion of the ankle. Moreover, the converging radii define a frustum that recreates the important triplanar motion of the ankle.

Another key design change is that the mobile-bearing concept was shifted from the implant to the instrumentation at the stage of tibial trial reduction. The instrumentation allows for a precise amount of bone resection from the tibia and talus that is equal to the overall thickness of the prosthesis (**Fig. 3**). The trial tibial base is placed with the talus and UHMWPE insert. The tibial base is smooth and is allowed to rotate with ankle motion. This rotation sets the proper axis for the prosthesis. Once the proper axis is set, the tibial keel is created. Before final placement of the tibial prosthesis, the UHMWPE insert is fixed to the tibial tray.

PREOPERATIVE CONSIDERATIONS

Imaging of the total ankle replacement candidate must evaluate several criteria: (1) the presence of degenerative change to the ankle and the subtalar and talonavicular joints; (2) limb and articular alignment on standing films (hindfoot alignment views are also important to evaluate if frontal plane deformity exists); (3) joint subluxation or incongruent articular deformity; (4) computed tomography (CT) scans are indicated for evaluate periarticular cysts and to further delineate degenerative changes in the subtalar and talonavicular joints; and (5) magnetic resonance (MR) imaging is used by the authors if avascular necrosis is suspected in the talus or distal tibial in cases of posttraumatic arthritis. Small amounts of avascular necrosis that can be resected

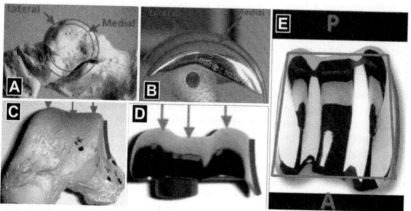

Fig. 2. Medial view of a cadaveric osseous model (*A*) and Salto Talaris talar component (*B*) and anterior view of a cadaveric osseous model (*C*) and Salto Talaris talar component (*D*) demonstrating the differing radii for the medial and lateral surfaces as is anatomically present in the human talus. Superior view of the Salto Talaris talar component (*E*) demonstrating the curvature to the differing radii and the wider aspect of the component being anterior as is anatomically present in the human talus (A, anterior; P, posterior).

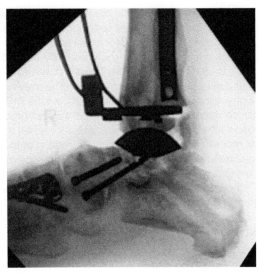

Fig. 3. Trial stage with talus and tibial tray in place. The tibial tray is allowed to rotate and translate with ankle motion. This is directed by the talus through the poly insert. The tibial tray must be seated properly before the keel is fashioned. The lateral C-arm view verifies proper posterior contact of the trial. Note the anterior slope has been reduced.

are of minimal consequence. Significant amounts of avascular necrosis may contraindicate a total ankle replacement.

Surgical Approach

The senior author (S.M.R.) has developed a perioperative protocol that is reproducible for all surgeons performing ankle replacement. All patients undergo a regional popliteal nerve block with catheter preoperatively in addition to general anesthesia. This has greatly improved pain control after the procedure and has also dramatically reduced the duration of hospital stays. A tourniquet is used for hemostasis to minimize blood loss. Generally, the procedure can be completed with less than 90 minutes of tourniquet time. After the prosthesis is placed, the tourniquet is released and hemostasis is assessed after irrigation before closure. Closure is performed over a reinfusion drain.

The procedure is performed with the patient in the supine position with a bump under the ipsilateral hip. The surgical incision is the standard approach for a total ankle procedure (interval between the extensor hallucis longus and the anterior tibial tendon). Throughout the procedure, proper handling of the anterior soft tissues is of upmost importance; wounds of the anterior compartment can be disastrous to manage. To minimize soft tissue damage, the author has adopted deep retraction with Gelphi retractors instead of skin-edge manual retraction to prevent necrosis. The periarticular osteophytes from the anterior distal aspect of the tibia and dorsal talar neck are removed. Resection of the anterior plafond must expose the apex of the plafond for accurate placement of the tibial alignment guide.[6]

Anterior Alignment Guide and Tibial Resection

The tibial alignment guide is zeroed and a pin is placed into the proximal tibia perpendicular to the anterior tibial tubercle (**Fig. 4**). The guide will then be aligned

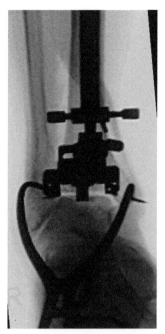

Fig. 4. Anterior alignment jig in place with talar alignment block. Note the coaxial alignment of the anatomic axis of the tibia and alignment guide. Deep retraction avoids skin edge necrosis. The talar alignment block is attached to align the prosthesis and talus.

to the tibial shaft (ie, anatomic axis) and secured distally with a medial pin. The guide and position relative to the tibial axis should be assessed with an intraoperative image intensification C-arm at this time. A useful modification at this step is to angle the proximal tibial pin inferior in the sagittal plane, removing the anterior slope of the tibial resection (**Fig. 5**). Removal of the anterior slope can improve motion postoperatively and protect from anterior subluxation in patients who have anterior talar listhesis (**Fig. 6**).

After the axial alignment has been confirmed, the distal alignment and proper size implant can be determined. Rotational alignment is set to the alignment of the talar body. Care must be taken with deformity that influences talar rotation. Varus hindfoot deformity will create external positioning of the talus. Internal malpositioning of the talar component will occur if the talar deformity is not recognized. Medial and lateral translation is used to fine-tune the tibial resection. The goal is to not resect the fibula and to leave enough medial isthmus on the malleolus to prevent iatrogenic fracture when placing the prosthesis. Medial and lateral positioning is adjusted to allow for the largest prosthesis without compromising the malleoli.

Initial tibial resection is no more than 9 mm from the roof of the plafond.

The tibial resection block is secured with medial and lateral shoulder pins and the plafond cut is made. The shoulder pins protect the malleoli during the tibial cut. Close clinical assessment must be taken at this step, because there may be rotational malalignment in the foot and tibia. Failure to recognize this malalignment will result in resecting too much posteromedial tibia or posterolateral fibula. The resected tibial bone is carefully removed to prevent malleolar fracture. The posterior malleolar fragment is safely left for removal after the posterior talar chamfer cut.

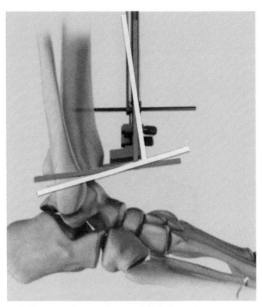

Fig. 5. Lateral view of illustrated osseous model demonstrating the traditional resection angle of the distal tibial plafond (*yellow line*) and the modification used to remove the anterior slope of the distal tibia (*orange line*).

Talar Bone Resection

The talar pin is set with the guide based off the tibial alignment guide and resection. The foot is held in a neutral position to accept the talar pin in the talus with the ankle in the functional neutral position. At this point, the tibial alignment guide can be

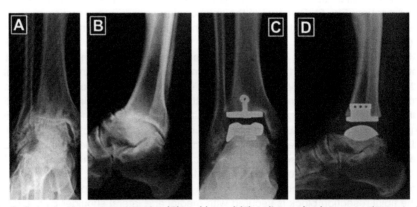

Fig. 6. Preoperative anteroposterior (*A*) and lateral (*B*) radiographs demonstrating anterior subluxation (listhesis) of the talus is associated with post-traumatic recurvatum articular deformity and chronic ankle instability. The talus must be repositioned beneath the tibial axis when the prosthesis is placed. Meticulous deltoid release and lateral ligament repair is often necessary to reestablish ligament stability. Postoperative anteroposterior (*C*) and lateral (*D*) radiographs following total ankle replacement. Note the anterior slope has been taken out to prevent anterior motion of the talus.

removed. The surgeon should leave the pins in place on the tibia. If additional bone is required, the cutting block can be replaced and additional resection preformed. With the talar pin in place, the posterior talar resection guide is placed with the paddles flush on the articular surface of the talus. The posterior talar chamfer cut is done carefully with care taken to protect the malleoli. With removal of the posterior talar dome, one can remove the remaining posterior distal aspect of the tibia.

Once the bone has been evacuated from the posterior tibia and the posterior chamfer resection is determined to be optimal, the remaining preparation can proceed. The anterior chamfer guide and resection is based off an accurate and precise posterior chamfer resection. The resection guide uses the anterior tibial plafond as a reference to ensure proper anterior to posterior positioning.

Trial Size Evaluation and Implant Selection

After bone resection, a thorough irrigation is helpful to remove debris and assess all resected surfaces for accuracy and completeness. The trial talus and tibia are placed. UHMWPE insert trials can be placed starting with 8-mm thickness to appropriately tension the collateral ligaments. In this important step, the surgeon must optimize conformity of the UHMWPE insert fit without binding motion in the prosthesis. Optimal motion may require lengthening of the posterior calf musculature during this step. At the same time as the proper size UHMWPE insert is chosen, the surgeon is performing a "dynamic flexion and extension" test. This allows the tibial tray to rotate and translate on the resected tibia. This motion is directed through the talus and UHMWPE insert. The author performs this sequence with lateral image intensification C-arm guidance. Proper seating of the tibial tray is critical at this step. Visual assessment of the tibial tray anteriorly and image intensification C-arm assessment of the posterior aspect of the tibial tray ensure proper position of the tibial tray on the resected tibial surface.

Once the proper size prosthesis and UHMWPE insert have been determined, and the functional axis of the prosthesis has been determined by dynamic motion, the keel can be prepared. Drilling of the keel sets the final position of the tibial component. Axial retrograde pressure on the foot is applied at this step. Once the keel is drilled and prepared, the trials are removed. The final UHMWPE is fixed to the tibial tray. The joint is irrigated of bone debris and the final prosthesis is inserted.

Several assessments must be determined at this time: (1) The implant must have uniform contact with the resected osseous surfaces. (2) The UHMWPE insert has optimal conformity without binding the ankle motion. Conversely, an undersized insert may inadequately tension the collateral ligaments that leads to unnecessary "slop" between the UHMWPE insert and talar component. (3) Make liberal use of intraoperative image intensification to evaluate the presence of malleolar fracture during implantation. (4) Hindfoot alignment should also be evaluated. Excessive varus of valgus mal-alignment will result in excessive eccentric loading and potential early prosthesis failure. (5) Bone grafting is performed of any cysts that were not included during osseous resection.

Deformity Evaluation and Surgical Considerations

The steps for bone resection are uniform for each individual procedure, although there are some key considerations to each deformity that must be evaluated and corrected with the surgical technique. Failure to evaluate and address intrinsic deformity will result in the prosthesis being placed without proper alignment, which can significantly alter the long-term prognosis of the prosthesis and UHMWPE insert.[7] Espinosa and colleagues[7] demonstrated that malalignment (>5°) of the prosthesis created UHMWPE contact pressures that exceeded the yield point in both fixed-bearing and mobile-bearing designs. This is an important concept, reinforcing that proper prosthesis alignment is critical regardless of whether a fixed or mobile-bearing device is used.

Bone loss or periarticular deformity can create deformity in any plane and presents with several considerations in ankle prosthesis. Careful preoperative planning will determine if the deformity can be corrected at the time of bone resection or if ancillary osteotomy is required. Often, asymmetric frontal plane bone loss can be corrected with simple bone resection. In general, the bone resection from the distal tibial plafond will correct intrinsic frontal plane bone loss. The proper bone resection is reliant on the anterior alignment jig being properly aligned in the frontal and sagittal plane.

Another consideration is periarticular bone cysts.[8] These are often identified radiographically and can be further delineated using preoperative CT scans (**Fig. 7**). Distal bone resection from the plafond usually eliminates any cyst formation. When the tibial bone resection does not remove periarticular cysts, grafting of the cyst becomes necessary.

There are instances when mechanical axis of the tibia is deviated in varus or, less often, valgus malalignment. The tibial alignment jig is designed to be placed parallel to the anatomic axis of the tibia. In these instances, the cutting jig should be aligned with the mechanical axis of the leg. This is defined as the center of the acetabulum to the center of the ankle joint.

Asymmetric bone loss from the talus results from various causes. The bone loss is usually associated with intrinsic varus or valgus malalignment. It is important to account for bone loss when making the talar cuts. This is done at the step of the posterior chamfer resection. Sheaths or "paddles" of various thicknesses can be placed over the posterior talar resection guide to account for this bone loss. Doing this ensures the plane of the posterior chamfer cut is parallel to the plafond resection in the frontal plane. Failure to do so will result in frontal plane malalignment of the talar prosthesis. This can potentially result in asymmetric tensioning of the collateral ligaments and frontal plane mal-alignment of the ankle and hindfoot.

Talar coverage is also important to achieve the best cortical overlap and fit of the prosthesis. The dimensions of the talar components are variable. The distance

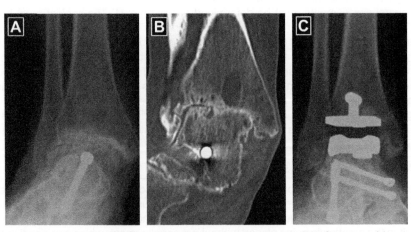

Fig. 7. Anteroposterior plain film (*A*) and coronal CT scan image (*B*) of 60-year-old woman with rheumatoid arthritis. Note the large plafond cyst, which was not resected with instrumentation during implantation of her Salto Talaris total ankle replacement (*C*). These bone defects must be grafted after placement of the final prosthesis.

between the center of the implant to the lateral flare of the talar component is fixed along all sizes. The medial width of the prosthesis is variable and can be sized up to appropriately cover the medial side of the talus. Further, the lateral chamfer cuts can be adjusted medially with small amounts for better medial bone coverage before performing the bell cut.

In instances with post-traumatic arthritis secondary to chronic ankle instability, the foot will drift anterior with respect to the mechanical axis of the tibia. The talus has been extruded anteriorly (talar listhesis). This lateral collateral ligament instability should be carefully evaluated in conjunction with varus malalignment. Reconstruction of the varus ankle has been well described by Schuberth and colleagues[9] to rebalance the intrinsically varus unstable ankle with arthroplasty. Deltoid sleeve release may be required in an effort to properly seat the talus posterior beneath the mechanical axis of the leg. In instances when the talus has been extruded forward, attempts at repositioning the talus back beneath the mechanical axis can result in fracture of the medial malleolus if appropriate soft tissue release has not been performed.

Clinical Results in the Salto Prosthesis

The Salto Talaris ankle implant has shown that patients have had success returning to activities without major complications. Bonnin and colleagues[5] in a prospective study evaluated 98 consecutive implants in 96 patients between 1997 and 2000. Ninety-three implants in 91 patients were available for review. Sixty-two women and 36 men with a mean age of 56 years were reported with a mean follow-up of 35 months. The overall survivorship of the Salto prosthesis at 68 months when using surgical revision or radiographic loosening as the end point was reported to be 93.8% in the favorable scenario and 91.8% in the unfavorable scenario, and using implant removal as the endpoint, the rates were 98% and 94.9%, respectively. In addition, mean American Orthopedic Foot and Ankle Society scores improved significantly from 32.3 points preoperatively to 83.1 points postoperatively. Dynamic range of motion radiographs also showed significant improvement from 15.2° preoperatively to 28.3° at follow-up. The authors concluded that these results were encouraging and supported the concept of anatomic replacement to improve functional outcomes but recognized the need for longer follow-up for further validation.

Bonin and colleagues[8] followed their original study with a survivorship analysis (7–11 years). They found that survival at 10 years without any reoperation was 65%. Six implants had to be converted to ankle arthrodesis. Other reasons for reoperation included UHMWPE insert exchange, symptomatic osteolytic cysts, and osteolysis. The authors concluded that there were 3 main reasons for reoperation: (1) bone cysts, (2) UHMWPE insert fracture, and (3) unexplained pain.

It should be noted that in all of these reports, and in the authors' practice, the Salto Talaris total ankle replacement is implanted without antibiotic polymethylmethacrylate cement fixation. The effect on implant longevity and patient outcomes with cement fixation is therefore unknown.

Range of Motion

Schuberth and colleagues[9] studied range of motion of the Salto Talaris during the first year of placement. Ninety-seven cases were examined at regular intervals at 6 weeks (11°) and at the 3-month (14°), 6-month (18°), and 12-month (20°) follow-ups. They demonstrated that motion increased the most between the 6-week and 6-month marks. The results of the study demonstrated that at least 20° of ankle motion can be expected after Salto Talaris implant arthroplasty at 1 year postoperatively.[9]

Leszko and colleagues[10] used fluoroscopy and 3 dimensional–to–2-dimensional registration techniques to determine the in vivo kinematics for 20 total ankle replacement subjects in performing 2 activities: gait and step-up. They witnessed translation of the mobile-bearing 1.5-mm and 2.3-mm devices for the 2 activities, respectively. From this data the authors concluded the dominant motion must be rotation.[10]

POSTOPERATIVE PROTOCOL

After implantation, the patient remains in the hospital for an average of 2 days. The drain is removed on postoperative day 2. Venous thromboembolism prophylaxis is initiated on postoperative day 1 and continued for 21 days. The patient is seen at 10 days; the sutures are removed, and the patient is placed in a below-the-knee non–weight-bearing cast. In general, the patient is non–weight bearing for 5 weeks, after which graduated weight bearing and physical therapy begin. In isolated cases, the patient is allowed early weight bearing in a cast at 3 weeks to assist is seating the prosthesis.

COMPLICATIONS

The general complications associated with the Salto Talaris ankle replacement prosthesis are the same as with other replacement systems. They can be categorized into soft tissue and prosthesis-related complications. Complications involved in the soft tissue are centered on wound healing and infection. Taking meticulous care of the anterior soft tissues during the surgery and avoiding skin edge retraction with manual retractors are critical in minimizing wound edge necrosis. Prevention of infection should be of primary importance to all surgeons performing total ankle replacement. The authors use a 3-day preoperative preparation with 4% weight/volume chlorhexidine gluconate scrub of the operated extremity before surgery. Preoperative antibiotics are indicated in all cases. Close attention should be paid to when the antibiotics are given; they should be given at least 1 hour before the operation to maximize soft tissue penetration. Maintenance of hemostasis and avoidance of undermining of the subcutaneous flaps are critical and maintaining the health and viability of the anterior soft tissue envelope. Skin closure should be performed in layers over a closed suction drain.

Prosthesis-related complications are highly variable. The most common reasons for implant revision and failure reported in the literature are the results of implant loosening, infection, and malalignment.[4,11] These complications will never be absolutely avoided, although close attention to surgical technique can mitigate avoidable errors. Close attention to proper size and fit of the prosthesis minimizes binding of the prosthesis and gutter impingement. Optimizing cortical overlap is critical to the long-term stability of the prosthesis (**Fig. 8**). Removal of osteophytes from the medial and lateral gutters also reduces the risk of impingement. Ensuring the prosthesis is properly seated on the tibia and talus is critical to the osseous on-growth of the implant. All bone cysts that are not resected must be grafted to ensure the best substrate for the prosthesis. Aseptic loosening and osteolysis have been reported and are difficult to predict. In general, it is agreed that this is caused by poor osseous ingrowth or UHMWPE insert particulate wear debris reactions. Mechanical factors also come in to play, such as poor alignment and eccentric loading of the implant, which can cause the implant to wear abnormally and eventually fail. Alignment is also critical to UHMWPE insert wear. Eccentric loading of the UHMWPE insert can cause early wear patterns and fracture (see **Fig. 8**).

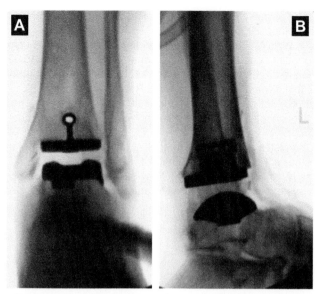

Fig. 8. Proper alignment of the total ankle replacement minimizes eccentric loading of the prosthesis. Optimizing cortical overlap and UHMWPE insert conformity with motion minimize edge loading of the insert.

SUMMARY

Total ankle replacement remains an evolving procedure to treat in stage ankle arthritis. The unique anatomy associated with the ankle, post-traumatic deformity, ligamentous instability, and variable bone quality makes ankle joint replacement a challenging endeavor. Close attention to the surgical technique and patient selection is critical to the ultimate success of the procedure. Further, understanding the surgical biomechanics associated with total ankle replacement and realignment of the foot is critical to the long-term success of the prosthesis. Recent results showing high clinical success and functional outcomes with total ankle replacement ensure that the new-generation prostheses will continue to be a valuable and predictable option for patients with end-stage ankle arthritis. The true role of polymethylmethacrylate cement fixation remains unknown, as no data exist comparing this with the off-label use of an uncemented Salto Talaris total ankle replacement in the United States.

REFERENCES

1. Chou LB, Coughlin MT, Hansen S Jr, et al. Osteoarthritis of the ankle: the role of arthroplasty. J Am Acad Orthop Surg 2008;16:249–59.
2. Piriou P, Culpan P, Mullins M, et al. Ankle replacement versus arthrodesis: a comparative gait analysis study. Foot Ankle Int 2008;29:3–9.
3. SooHoo NF, Zingmond DS, Lo CY. Comparison of reoperation rates following ankle arthrodesis and total ankle arthroplasty. J Bone Joint Surg Am 2007;89: 2143–9.
4. Cracchiola A 3rd, DeOrio JK. Design features of current total ankle replacments: implants and instrumentation. J Am Acad Orthop Surg 2008;16:530–40.
5. Bonin M, Judet T, Colombier JA, et al. Midterm results of the Salto total ankle prosthesis. Clin Orthop Relat Res 2004;424:6–18.

6. Yalamanchili P, Donely B, Casillas M, et al. Salto Talaris total ankle replacement. Oper Tech Orthop 2008;18:277–81.
7. Espinosa N, Walti M, Farve P, et al. Misalignment of total ankle components can induce high joint contact pressures. J Bone Joint Surg Am 2010;92:1179–87.
8. Bonin M, Gaudot F, Laurent J, et al. Salto total ankle arthroplasty survivorship and analysis 7 to 11 years. Clin Orthop Relat Res 2010;469:225–36.
9. Schuberth JS, McCourt MJ, Christensen JC. Interval changes in postoperative range of motion of Salto Talaris total ankle replacement. J Foot Ankle Surg 2011;50:562–5.
10. Leszko F, Komistek RD, Mahfouz MR, et al. In vivo kinematics of the Salto total ankle prosthesis. Foot Ankle Int 2008;29:1117–25.
11. Gougoulias N, Khanna A, Maffulli N. How successful are current ankle replacements? A systematic review of the literature. Clin Orthop Relat Res 2010;468:199–208.

Agility to INBONE
Anterior and Posterior Approaches to the Difficult Revision Total Ankle Replacement

J. George DeVries, DPM, AACFAS[a], Ryan T. Scott, DPM, AACFAS[b],
Gregory C. Berlet, MD[b],*, Christopher F. Hyer, DPM, MS[b],
Thomas H. Lee, MD[b], James K. DeOrio, MD[c]

KEYWORDS

- Total ankle replacement • Revision • INBONE • Agility

KEY POINTS

- The options for salvage of a failed Agility total ankle replacement are technically demanding and require careful consideration both from the surgeon and the patient.
- The INBONE total ankle replacement is an excellent revision ankle replacement, because of its modularity and the ability to make up any tibial bone loss.
- Salvage of a failed Agility total ankle replacement by conversion to INBONE total ankle replacement can be accomplished, although the risk of complication or failure is very high.
- The surgeons must properly educate their patients about the potential complications with revision total ankle replacement including further revisions, gutter decompression, conversion to tibio-talo-calcaneal arthrodesis, or even below-the-knee amputation.

INTRODUCTION

Total ankle replacement has been gaining acceptance since the introduction of second-generation and third-generation implants. Subspecialty orthopedic foot and ankle surgeons surveyed by the American Orthopedic Foot and Ankle Surgeons had an adoption rate of 51.0% in 2004 and 63.5% in 2012, whereas overall adoption rate within foot and ankle care providers was noted to be 30%.[1,2] This expansion is partly because of better technique and instrumentation, but also an expansion of indications. Early contraindications, such as varus and valgus deformity are now being overcome

The authors, Drs Berlet, Lee, DeOrio, and Hyer, are consultants for Wright Medical Technology, Inc. Dr DeVries serves as educational faculty with Arthrex, Inc.

[a] Excel Orthopedics, 705 South University Avenue, Suite 150, Beaver Dam, WI 53916, USA; [b] Orthopedic Foot and Ankle Center, 300 Polaris Parkway, Suite 2000, Westerville, OH 43082, USA; [c] Department of Orthopedics, Duke University, Duke Medical Plaza, Suite 200, 4709 Creekstone Drive, Durham, NC 27703, USA

* Corresponding author. Orthopedic Foot and Ankle Center, 300 Polaris Parkway, Suite 2000, Westerville, OH 43082.

E-mail address: ofacresearch@orthofootankle.com

Clin Podiatr Med Surg 30 (2013) 81–96
http://dx.doi.org/10.1016/j.cpm.2012.08.011   **podiatric.theclinics.com**
0891-8422/13/$ – see front matter © 2013 Elsevier Inc. All rights reserved.

as surgeons gain experience with this procedure, different constraints within newer prostheses, and more refined techniques of ligament rebalancing.[3,4] As more challenging cases are addressed with total ankle replacement, adjunct procedures during and following prosthetic implantation will become more common. It may be that total ankle replacement is best thought of as a continuum and not an isolated surgery.

Failure of a total ankle replacement is a challenging problem to both the patient and surgeon, offering a very difficult decision on whether revision or fusion is the more viable option. The bony resection required for revision may be increased if the failed total ankle replacement had aseptic osteolysis around the components, with or without implant loosening. In 2 studies examining the Agility total ankle replacement (DePuy Orthopedics, Inc, Warsaw, IN), the incidence of osteolysis was 76% to 85%, although this did not necessarily lead to complications or implant failure.[5,6] A large retrospective analysis of complications and failure in the Agility total ankle replacement found an overall failure rate of 10.8%, with failure defined as component revision, salvage arthrodesis, or below-knee amputation.[7]

Several studies have evaluated the Scandinavian Total Ankle Replacement (STAR) (Small Bone Innovations, Inc, Morrisville, PA). Valderrabano and colleagues[8] in 2004 found 3 instances of ballooning lysis around the tibial component. They also noted that 43 ankles had hypertrophic bone formation around the ankle joint in a study of 68 STAR Ankles. They noted 9 revision total ankle replacements at an average of 3.7 years postoperative. A study by Wood and Deakin in 2008[9] found that there were 25 ankles with aseptic loosening in a group of 200 prospectively followed STAR ankles. Overall, 4 were revised, 1 required bone grafting owing to talar subsidence, and 10 ankles required arthrodesis.

The salvage options for failed total ankle replacement are scantily reported in the literature, and all are technically demanding. Arthrodesis is frequently reported as the "gold standard" as a primary and secondary salvage option. Arthrodesis is typically performed using a combination of screws and plates, or a retrograde compression locked intramedullary nail with bulk allograft bone grafting.[10–12] Revision options, including ultra-high molecular weight polyethylene (UHMWPE) insert exchange with or without removal and substitution of the metallic components has also been reported with success for early total ankle replacement failure.[7]

There are a few reports in the literature of converting an original total ankle replacement to a different design. Myerson and Won[13] discuss the role of a custom-designed, stemmed implant for both primary and revision total ankle replacement; however, no results have been reported. Kharwadkar and Harris[14] reported 2 cases of the conversion of failed STAR to a hybrid of systems using components from the Ankle Evolution System (AES) (Biomet Germany, Berlin, Germany) and the STAR. Assal and colleagues[15] and DiDomenico and Williams[16] reported the conversion of a modified Buechel-Pappas Total Ankle System (Endotec, Inc, South Orange, NJ) to an Agility total ankle replacement. The unique design of Agility, with its wide tibial base, made this implant uniquely suited for revision replacement of a failed implant.

Although conversion total ankle replacement through the previous anterior incision is an intuitive approach, occasionally this approach will not be possible. Wound complications using the utilitarian anterior incision are frequently reported in the literature with rates of wound complications ranging from 2.0% to 20.9%.[9,17–22] Major wound complications requiring soft tissue coverage occur in 1% to 2% of cases.[9,19,20] These complications, requiring skin grafting, rotation flaps, or free tissue transfer, make the anterior approach undesirable or impossible for revision total ankle replacement.

The open posterior approach to the ankle joint has seldom been described in the literature. Hanson and Cracchiolo[23] originally discussed the posterior approach and applications of a 95° blade plate as an alternative for tibio-talo-calcaneal arthrodesis in 10 patients. Seven of the 10 patients had previous ankle or hindfoot surgery, but none through a posterior approach. Three of the patients had complications: 1 transient neuropraxia, 1 wound complication, and 1 deep venous thrombosis.

The authors of the current article describe the technique for both the anterior and posterior approach to revision Agility total ankle replacement by conversion to the INBONE total ankle replacement (Wright Medical Technologies, Memphis, TN) implant. This offers versatility and modularity for conversion of the failed total ankle replacement. In the case series, the authors present 13 patients who have been converted from an Agility total ankle replacement to an INBONE total ankle replacement through an anterior approach, followed for a minimum of 6 months. In addition, a single case of the posterior approach conversion is reported.

Surgical Technique

Anterior approach

The patient is placed on the operating table in the supine position and general anesthesia is induced. For convenience, the contralateral leg may be placed into a thigh holder to allow for access to the operative leg with an intraoperative image intensification C-arm. The operative leg is scrubbed, prepped, and draped to the mid-thigh. A thigh tourniquet is used for hemostasis. A minimally invasive incision is placed through the previous anterior approach between the extensor hallucis longus and the tibialis anterior tendons. The extensor retinaculum is tagged during initial dissection as the scar formation during revision total ankle replacement may make identification of the retinaculum difficult after reimplantation. The original implant is then visualized. Removal of all fibrotic scarring, or heterotrophic ossification is performed allowing for visualization of the original implant.

Using curettes and ronguers carefully identify the interface between the host bone and implant. The order for implant removal is poly, tibia, and then talus. This is done to remove as little host bone as possible (**Fig. 1**A).

The UHMWPE insert component is removed first, either in toto or piecemeal. A 0.25-inch osteotome can be used between the metal and UHMWPE insert components medially and laterally to removed the interlocking portion of the polyethylene insert. The UHMWPE can then be pried distally off the metal tibial component and removed. The other choice is to use the sagittal saw and cut the columns off the UHMWPE insert.

The tibia is the biggest challenge and the one in which most time will be spent. The anterior distal tibia is resected down to the tibial component to expose the distal tibial-implant interface. Prophylactic pinning with guide wires for cannulated screws and/or insertion of fully threaded screws should be carried out before implant extraction. This step can be achieved quickly and is universally used by the authors for these complex cases. To remove the original implant, use either fine oscillating and/or reciprocal saws to cut the prosthesis away from bony or fibrous ingrowth. Using saws, instead of osteotomes, may help save as much bone as possible and help avoid fractures. The proximal stem of the original implant must be freed, and may require a small cortical window. In most cases, the Agility total ankle replacement stem can be delivered distally without the need for an anterior cortical window. Care must be taken to preserve the structural integrity of the anterior distal tibial cortex as much as possible; however, the intramedullary stem of the INBONE total ankle replacement with added segments will help account for any loss of bone integrity distally. The Agility implant is then carefully explanted with gentle manipulation to avoid fracture of the malleoli. Because the distal anterior cortex of the tibia will support the tibial component, if it

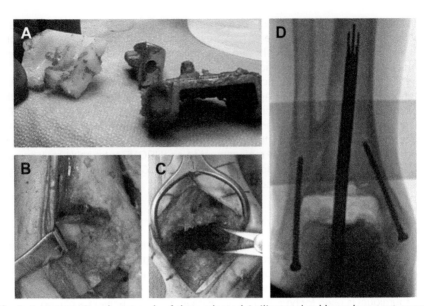

Fig. 1. Intraoperative photograph of the explanted Agility total ankle replacement components (*A*). Photograph demonstrating the osseous void after Agility total ankle replacement removal (*B*). A laminar spreader is useful in helping to make sure there is an end point of both the medial and lateral ligaments (*C*). Anterior-posterior intraoperative image intensification view demonstrating intramedullary alignment for implantation of the INBONE total ankle replacement (*D*). Note the prophylactic bimalleolar screw fixation for structural support.

is missing, when the patient applies weight on the ankle the prosthesis will go into flexion. To avoid this problem if present, an allograft bone graft will need to be inset anteriorly to prevent the prosthesis from flexion or up to 4 or 5 extra segments of tibial components of the stem will need to be added to keep the prosthesis from flexing excessively. We prefer the allograft bone graft technique.

Once the tibial component is removed, attention is directed to the talar component. Because the amount of bone left in the talus is critical, the use of the fine saws is crucial. Only after you have reached the extent of the saw should you move to the use of an osteotome or periosteal elevator and remove the Agility prosthesis. Solid porous ingrowth of the talus is relatively uncommon. Attention is paid to the condition of the talus, evaluating for cystic changes, and particular attention should be directed to the medial and lateral gutters (see **Fig. 1**B). The gutters are decompressed of any impinging soft tissue or osseous structures, with care taken to maintain adequate bone stock for the talar implant. Any remaining hardware that will inhibit implantation of the INBONE total ankle replacement is removed. This can often be done at the beginning of the case as well, with the tourniquet down to save tourniquet time. Finally, the soft tissue structures are then examined for an end point both medially and laterally, giving an insight into whether or not ligament rebalancing will be required. This can be evaluated by using a laminar spreader to distract longitudinally checking for end point on both the medial and lateral sides (see **Fig. 1**C).

After soft tissue balancing, removal of the original implant, and adequate decompression of the gutters, the foot is placed into the leg holder for subsequent implantation of the INBONE total ankle replacement. Obtaining a mortise view can be difficult after all resection has taken place, in which case the foot may be loaded into the jig with the medial malleolar axis parallel to the foot plate. The space between the tibia and remaining talus may be maintained with either lamina spreaders or Steinmann pins. Once proper positioning has been obtained, the calcaneus is pinned to the jig. Accurate positioning for the intramedullary drill is obtained using the targeting guides (see **Fig. 1**D). The drill is then advanced through the calcaneus, talus, and into the tibia.

The appropriate INBONE total ankle replacement trial sizer is selected for the revision replacement. This is selected based on the medial-to-lateral width of the distal tibia, understanding that lateral ballooning osteolysis from the Agility total ankle replacement will often remove the lateral side as an effective point of reference. Care must be taken to avoid or minimally resect the medial malleolus, while avoiding the lateral malleolus entirely. Lateral view sizing is also done preoperatively to determine anterior to posterior coverage and stem placement. Normally, the joint line determines the distal to proximal positioning of the tibial and talar cuts; however, these references may be distorted or absent in the case of revision total ankle replacement. Thus, the references that are used in revision surgery are different relative to the previous native joint line. On the mortise view, the medial-to-lateral resection is determined via the distal, widest portion of the cut guide. Attention is directed to ensure that any further resection of the malleoli will not occur, and no overhang of the talar component is identified. Oversizing the talus could cause impingement with the malleoli. On the lateral view, the talar cut is determined by placing 2 saw blades into the cut guide. Lamina spreaders again may be used at this point to distract the tibia and talus to avoid resecting too much bone, particularly if there has been significant subsidence. This also allows the surgeon to identify and create the new joint line. The cut margins should ideally be just grazing the top of the talus, and also providing minimal tibia resection.

Joint line restoration is important for ankle kinematics. The joint line is almost always elevated because of tibial bone loss. The joint line can be reestablished by using either a larger UHMWPE insert or moving the tibial base plate inferiorly with bone grafting between the host bone and the new tibial base plate. Using a larger UHMWPE insert is the preferred option of these.

Any large cysts or defects within the tibia or talus that are contained need to be packed with graft. Because minimal bone is resected in these revision cases, allograft bone is often used.

After proper positioning and sizing, the implantation follows standard surgical technique with close attention being paid to proximal fixation of the INBONE tibial stem. Once both the tibia and talus implants have been placed, trial UHMWPE insert sizes are used while final soft tissue balancing is performed. Any other reconstructive procedures, such as tendon transfers, calcaneal osteotomy, ligament reconstruction, gastrocnemius recession, and midfoot/hindfoot arthrodesis, may be performed at this point as necessary to attain a balanced ankle. Avoid overstuffing the joint, as too much tension may lead to a stiff joint, with reduced range of motion postoperatively. Ensure that at least a minimal range of motion is attained, although this may be less than desired depending on the range the patient had preoperatively. You may encounter a case where, because of extensive bone loss, stability cannot be achieved in the ankle because the UHMWPE insert width stops at 14 mm. In this instance, the authors have made, out of a femoral head, a tricortical "collar" and placed this at the distal end of the tibia between the base plate of the prosthesis and the tibia. Additional bone graft is then added as needed.

The wound is thoroughly irrigated and closed in layers. Particular attention is given to a strong retinaculum closure to prevent bowstringing of the extensor tendons. The patient is placed into a splint or cast according to surgeon preference, and is non–weight bearing for 4 weeks. Protected weight bearing and range of motion may be instituted at 4 weeks as long as there are no wound complications.

Posterior approach

This novel approach may be considered in the face of previous anterior wound complications that preclude standard anterior incisional approaches and its use would be only under extraordinary circumstances (**Fig. 2**). The method presented here was accomplished by one of the authors (T.H.L.) with custom jigs inserted freehand and the ankle inserted in reverse.

The patient is placed on the operating table in the prone position and general anesthesia is induced. The operative leg is scrubbed and prepped to the mid-thigh, and a thigh tourniquet is used for hemostasis. A 15-cm longitudinal incision is used. Dissection is carried down to the Achilles tendon, which is then split longitudinally, leaving it intact or performing a Z-lengthening. The portions of the exposed tendon are kept moist throughout the procedure. Dissection is then continued midline to the flexor hallucis longus fascia and muscle belly. The muscle belly is elevated with a periosteal elevator and retracted medially, along with the posterior tibial neurovascular bundle. The posterior fibula is now just posterior and lateral to the tibia, and the flexor hallucis longus muscle belly and neurovascular bundle are posterior and medial to the tibia. The posterior ankle capsule is then exposed and opened midline. Any remaining posterior malleolus is removed, along with excessive arthrofibrosis and heterotrophic ossification. The original implant is then visualized (**Fig. 3A**).

Explantation of the original components through a posterior approach progresses along a similar set of steps as used for the anterior approach. The UHMWPE insert is removed first, again either in toto or piecemeal. The posterior-inferior tibia is then removed minimally at the tibial-implant interface. Any stems of the original implant

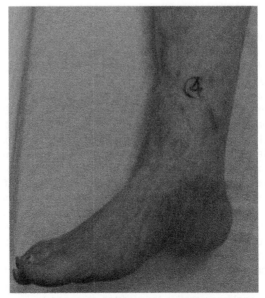

Fig. 2. Clinical photograph demonstrating free tissue transfer well incorporated about the anterior ankle, posing concern for wound complications during subsequent revision total ankle replacement.

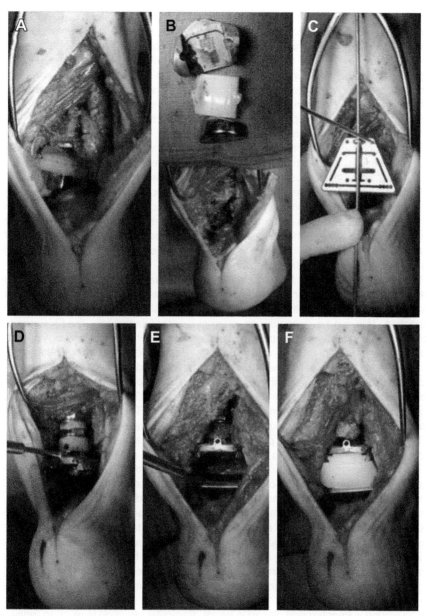

Fig. 3. Posterior approach with a Z-style Achilles tendon split demonstrating posterior exposure of the failed Agility total ankle replacement (*A*) that is then removed (*B*). Photograph demonstrating technique to identify the extramedullary tibial axis, while using the cutting guide (*C*). Implantation of the INBONE total ankle replacement tibial stem and tray components (*D*). Note the removal of the posterior distal tibial cortical window to allow for replacement insertion. Implantation of the talar component (*E*) and UHMWPE insert (*F*). Note the placement of the posterior distal tibial cortical window back into place to cover tibial component. Additionally, recognize that the INBONE total ankle replacement components have been inserted "backward."

are taken into account and may require some posterior wall removal. The tibial component is then removed. Once the tibial component is removed, the talar component is removed much the same way as during the anterior approach. The talus again must be inspected for any loss of mass or structure, and will have to be addressed (see **Fig. 3B**). Any remaining hardware that will impede the new implantation is removed. A mortise view is important to obtain for proper reference; however, when no jig is used, the view will be changing constantly. Nonetheless, the mortise is more readily conceptualized during the posterior approach, as the fibula, which projects posterior to the tibia, is largely exposed into the operative field.

The cutting guides used for this posterior approach were custom guides, which do not require the jig. Instead they rely on an extramedullary guide pin that can be placed on the tibia, with position confirmed using a mortise view (see **Fig. 3C**). Positioning is determined in much the same way as for the anterior approach. The distal to proximal positioning again is determined to ensure minimal resection at both the tibial and talar levels, but the talar neck is not available as a reference. Instead, positioning is determined by placing the foot in a rectus position, and resection of all cystic or structurally unsound bone is undertaken. Once the guide position is determined, the cutting guide is pinned into place using the incorporated pinholes.

The bone resection then takes place, and the resected bone is removed. The intramedullary reaming used for the standard technique can be done, but the entire tibio-talo-calcaneal complex will need to be stabilized to allow for accurate reaming and impaction. This can be done with an external fixator. Alternatively, the tibial component can be implanted backward through a posterior cortical window, similar to the standard anterior implantation of the Buechel-Pappas total ankle replacement[24] or some custom-designed total ankle replacements, as described by Myerson and Won.[13] The medullary canal of the distal tibia is curetted to accommodate the implant, and the implant is placed within the ankle (see **Fig. 3D**). The cortical window is then placed back over the tibial stem and secured into place. This can be done with either plates and screws, or simple suture with sound soft tissue coverage.

The talar component can be placed with reaming over a guide pin as with standard technique. Again, without the jig and intramedullary guide, placement is based on tibial component placement and mortise positioning of the ankle. The guide pin is inserted centered under the tibial component. The guide pin is inserted at 45° of angulation to the cut surface of the talus and the reamer is advanced over it. Once the canal is reamed, the talar component can be inserted in reverse (see **Fig. 3E**). The bone under the talar component may need bone grafting or packing to augment the loss of bone from the original failed total ankle replacement. Alternatively, a subtalar joint arthrodesis of the posterior facet may allow for increased bony fixation. Once the tibial and talar components are stable, the polymer can be inserted using the standard technique, again making sure it is facing posteriorly, consistent with the other components (see **Fig. 3F**).

The wound is irrigated and closed in layers. Particular attention is given to repairing the longitudinal opening or Z-lengthening of the Achilles tendon into physiologic tension. The patient is placed into a splint or cast according to surgeon preference, and is non–weight bearing for 4 to 6 weeks. Protected weight bearing and range of motion may be instituted at that point as long as there are no wound complications.

PATIENTS AND METHODS

All patients who had a revision of a failed Agility total ankle replacement by conversion to an INBONE total ankle replacement between September 2007 and December 2011 and have been followed a minimum of 6 months were included. A single patient was converted through a posterior approach. All surgeries were performed by 1 of 3 senior authors (G.C.B., T.H.L., J.K.D.) at both the Orthopedic Foot and Ankle Center in Ohio or Duke University in North Carolina. All patients experienced continued pain and or deformity and were extensively counseled on the risks and benefits of conversion to revision total ankle replacement. Data were gathered using retrospective chart review. Outcomes and complications were recorded. Complications were considered major if they required a secondary operative intervention, and minor if there were changes that did not require a secondary surgery. The authors will also highlight several specific cases.

RESULTS

A total of 14 patients met inclusion criteria and were available for review. Thirteen patients were converted through an anterior approach, and a single patient was converted through a posterior approach. The average age at the time of the conversion was 65.2 ± 11.5 years (range, 45–79 years). There were 8 men (57.1%) and 6 women. No patients were active smokers at the time of conversion, although 5 patients (35.7%) did admit to a previous history of smoking. The patients presented with a variety of past medical problems and included 3 patients (21.4%) who were diabetic. The average follow-up was 2.4 ± 1.4 years (range, 7 months to 4.6 years).

The original Agility total ankle replacement had been in place an average of 7.8 ± 4.8 years (range, 3.5–23.0 years), and most were implanted owing to primary or posttraumatic osteoarthritis. One patient had rheumatoid arthritis. Osteolysis and aseptic loosening were the most common reasons for failure. The average size of the tibial and talar INBONE total ankle replacement components placed was 3.8 ± 0.9 (size 3 to size 6). The average UHMWPE insert thickness was 11.9 ± 2.4 mm (range, 8–15 mm). All patients had some adjunctive procedure done at the time of the conversion, from simple hardware removal to concomitant subtalar joint arthrodesis. Patients progressed to partial or protected weight bearing at 5.6 ± 1.4 weeks (range, 3–8 weeks) and then to full weight bearing at 8.7 ± 1.4 weeks (range, 6–12 weeks).

Overall, 9 patients (64.3%) had complications. There were 5 major complications (35.7%) that required a secondary operative intervention. This involved 1 plantar neurolysis, 1 wound incision and drainage, and 1 UHMWPE insert exchange with concomitant lateral ankle stabilization. There were 2 cases that had major complications that were considered failures. One patient had a history of minor wound complications after the original Agility total ankle replacement. He then developed a deep infection after placement of the INBONE total ankle replacement that was treated with incision and drainage and an antibiotic-loaded polymethylmethacrylate cement spacer that was salvaged with a tibio-talo-calcaneal arthrodesis fixated with a retrograde locked compression intramedullary nail and femoral head allograft. One patient, the oldest in the series, developed a wound complication that led to a deep-seated infection. He was ultimately treated with a below-the-knee amputation. There were also 4 minor complications (28.6%), and included some asymptomatic component subsidence and some residual pain.

HIGHLIGHTED CASE STUDIES
Case 1

A 74-year-old woman with a past medical history of diabetes, hypertension, asthma, and basal cell carcinoma of the scalp presented to our office with drainage from her right ankle 4 years status post original Agility total ankle replacement (**Fig. 4**A, B).

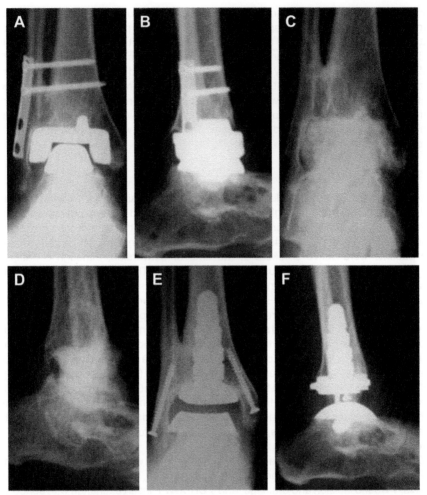

Fig. 4. Anterior-posterior (*A*) and lateral (*B*) radiographs of an infected Agility total ankle replacement. Anterior-posterior (*C*) and lateral (*D*) radiographs following insertion of an antibiotic-loaded polymethylmethacrylate cement spacer after explantation of the Agility total ankle replacement. Anterior-posterior (*E*) and lateral (*F*) radiographs demonstrating conversion to an INBONE total ankle replacement with prophylactic bimalleolar screw fixation.

The patient did undergo multiple irrigation and débridement, as well as a hardware removal of the syndesmotic screws and UHMWPE insert exchange before presentation to the authors. At 6 years after the index total ankle replacement, the patient presented to the emergency department with pain and a red, hot swollen ankle with purulent discharge expressing through the lateral wound with range of motion. Immediate explantation of the total ankle replacement and insertion of an antibiotic-loaded polymethylmethacrylate cement spacer was performed (see **Fig. 4**C, D). The patient was placed on intravenous antibiotics and serial inflammatory markers were followed until they normalized. Conversion total ankle replacement was performed 3 months later when no growth was identified on culture. The patient underwent explantation of the cement spacer, and placement of a size 3 tibial tray, 4-component tibial stem construct, 10-mm UHMWPE insert, and size 3 talar component with 10-mm stem.

Prophylactic percutaneous screw placement was used for "rebar" in both malleoli (see **Fig. 4**E, F). Postoperative course was uneventful. She was placed into an aggressive course of physical therapy and is doing well today. She is currently 21 months conversion total ankle replacement.

Case 2

Case 2 was a 68-year-old man with no significant past medical history complaining of pain and discomfort to his left ankle during ambulation following a previous Agility total ankle replacement. He initially underwent an Agility total ankle replacement secondary to posttraumatic degenerative joint disease from a previous ankle fracture (**Fig. 5**A, B).

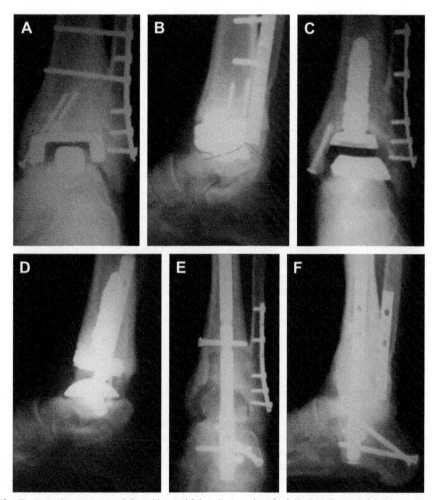

Fig. 5. Anterior-posterior (*A*) and lateral (*B*) radiographs of a failed Agility total ankle replacement. Anterior-posterior (*C*) and lateral (*D*) radiographs following conversion to an INBONE total ankle replacement. Anterior-posterior (*E*) and lateral (*F*) radiographs following explantation of the failed INBONE total ankle replacement and conversion to tibio-talo-calcaneal arthrodesis with bulk femoral head allograft using a retrograde compression locked intramedullary nail. (*From* DeVries JG, Berlet GC, Lee TH, et al. Revision total ankle replacement: an early look at agility to INBONE. Foot Ankle Spec 2011;4(4):235–44; with permission.)

He elected to undergo conversion total ankle replacement 3.5 years later because of pain, and the patient had heterotopic ossification of the original implant, a history of infection. The patient underwent explantation of the original Agility total ankle replacement and placement of a size 3 tibial tray, 5-component tibial stem construct, 8-mm UHMWPE insert, and size 3 talar component with 14-mm stem. He also had prophylactic percutaneous screw placement in the medial malleolus (see **Fig. 5**C, D). The postoperative course was complicated with an abscess over the anterior ankle. Multiple irrigation and débridement procedures were performed with application of negative pressure wound therapy. Explantation of the INBONE total ankle replacement was performed 14 months later with insertion of an antibiotic-loaded polymethylmethacrylate cement spacer. Serial inflammatory markers were followed until they normalized and there was no longer evidence of infection. A tibio-talo-calcaneal arthrodesis with femoral head allograft was then performed 17 months following the conversion total ankle replacement (see **Fig. 5**D, E). The patient is currently 2.5 years out from the tibio-talo-calcaneal arthrodesis and is doing well, back playing golf.

Case 3

Case 3 was a 70-year-old man with past medical history of hypertension, atrial fibrillation, deep vein thrombosis with pulmonary embolism, history of transient ischemic attack, and obstructive sleep apnea. Original Agility total ankle replacement was placed in 1999 with a UHMWPE exchange 1 year later (**Fig. 6**A, B). After his index operation, the patient suffered an anterior wound dehiscence, which required free flap coverage. Conversion total ankle replacement was performed 10 years after initial implant (9 years following UHMWPE exchange) secondary to aseptic loosening and pain. This procedure was performed via a posterior approach through a Z-style Achilles tenotomy. The patient underwent explantation of the original Agility total ankle replacement, talectomy with bone grafting, and placement of a size 4 tibial tray, 3-component tibial stem construct, 15-mm UHMWPE insert, and a size 4 talar component with 10-mm stem (see **Fig. 6**C, D). At 1.5 months postoperative, the patient underwent irrigation and débridement of the Achilles tendon and application of negative pressure wound therapy because of surgical wound dehiscence. The wound went on to heal without any further complications. He is currently 32 months out from conversion total ankle replacement and is ambulating without a brace and has no complaints.

DISCUSSION

The Agility total ankle replacement has been said to be better capable of dealing with bone loss by structurally resurfacing a larger portion of the joint when compared with previous generations of total ankle replacement.[15] This helped to influence the use of the Agility total ankle replacement in the management of ankle degenerative joint disease. Criswell and colleagues[25] noted that after 8 years of follow-up, 16 (39%) of their 42 Agility total ankle replacements required revision. Labek and colleagues[26] reported similar data following performing a literature search on revision surgery of the 6 most common total ankle replacement systems. Of the 6 studies, 682 patients were identified and 218 (32%) of the 682 required revision. On average, the revision was required 7.3 years postoperatively.

The authors of the present study chose to convert failed Agility total ankle replacements to INBONE total ankle replacements for several reasons. First, the modular tibial stem allows for stability and bony ingrowth on the prosthesis with less reliance on the distal tibial surface via load sharing. The wide resection into the malleoli needed

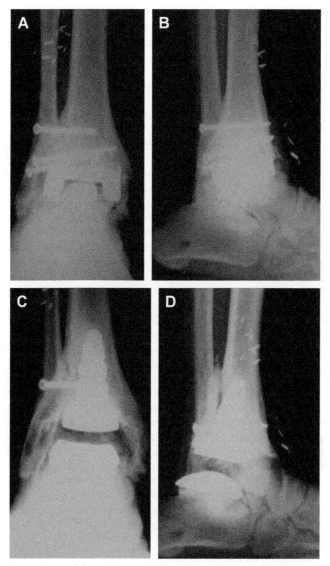

Fig. 6. Anterior-posterior (*A*) and lateral (*B*) radiographs of a failed Agility total ankle replacement. Note the staples from free tissue transfer about the anterior ankle. Anterior-posterior (*C*) and lateral (*D*) radiographs following posterior approach to implantation of the INBONE total ankle replacement demonstrated in **Fig. 3**. Note tibial tray and talar stem inserted "backward."

for the Agility total ankle replacement makes conversion to a different model of total ankle replacement difficult, whereas the INBONE total ankle replacement relies on the intramedullary canal for stability. Second, the most common form of failure of the Agility total ankle replacement the authors have encountered is talar subsidence. The INBONE total ankle replacement offers a very wide talar base, which is useful for securing maximal support for the remaining talus, as well as offering a wide base for bone graft back filling. Third, the INBONE total ankle replacement offers modularity of the porous-coated talar component, as well, with both short (10 mm) and long (14 mm) talar stems. Fourth, the INBONE total ankle replacement offers UHMWPE inserts up to 15 mm to help accommodate some of the excessive bony loss in revision total ankle replacement. This allows some accommodation by lowering the revision joint line to the more native ankle joint. Fifth, the jig used for implantation of the INBONE total ankle replacement allows for reproducible installation of the components. This can be especially beneficial in revision total ankle replacement, as the normal anatomy is often distorted, potentially leading to malorientation of the components. An improperly positioned ankle is doomed to failure.

The posterior approach to conversion to INBONE total ankle replacement may be a possibility for patients requiring revision. It should be emphasized that this is not to be taken as a recommendation of the technique, just a possible future direction. A holder designed for posterior positioning is not currently available, but could potentially expand the ability to convert failed total ankle replacements to INBONE total ankle replacements. So too could the new Prophecy technique (Prophecy INBONE Pre-Operative Navigation Alignment Guide, Wright Medical Technology, Arlington, TN) be used for a posterior approach. This technique is just being introduced, in which plastic blocks are made preoperatively based on a computed tomography scan and the leg holder is not used.

The implantation of the total ankle replacement in reverse is counterintuitive, but functionally is an option because the patient may retain some motion. The talar component has a few attributes that allow this approach. First, the UHMWPE insert and the talar component are contoured to match each other in a close fit. This allows for stability regardless of the directionality, as long as both components are placed in the same direction. Second, the talar component is anatomically designed to be slightly narrower posterior than anterior. Thus, when a patient with a reversed implant dorsiflexes, the ankle will have less inherent constraint. Although this could be a problem for a primary total ankle in a patient in whose motion is sufficient, this is not the case in revision total ankle replacement. Range of motion is most often severely decreased in patients requiring revision total ankle replacement. Therefore, this reduced constraint with dorsiflexion may allow for maximal motion. The fixed bearing design of the INBONE total ankle replacement will allow this reverse-facing implant to maintain stability. And, finally, when the implant is placed in reverse, the talar stem actually projects anteriorly as opposed to posteriorly, as in the standard approach. This will allow for the stem to go toward the talar neck as opposed to the posterior facet, and may accommodate a longer stem than what otherwise would have to be used.

SUMMARY

As total ankle replacement continues to grow in popularity and the indications are expanded, the number of revisions required is likely to increase. The options for salvage are all technically demanding and require careful consideration, both from the surgeon and the patient. Total ankle replacement conversion is minimally discussed in the literature. The authors have shown that salvage of a failed Agility total ankle replacement by conversion to INBONE total ankle replacement can be accomplished, although the risk of complication or failure is very high. The surgeons must properly educate their patients about the potential complications with revision total ankle replacement, including further revisions, gutter decompression, conversion to tibio-talo-calcaneal arthrodesis, or even below-the-knee amputation. Although this case series has all the weaknesses inherent to a case series, including no prospective data and the potential of bias in reporting, the authors believe this to be valuable information to any foot and ankle surgeon faced with a failed total ankle replacement.

REFERENCES

1. Eisner W. New survey reveals top foot and ankle suppliers. Orthopedics This Week. (Week 8) 2012.
2. Lau JTC, Schon LC, Mahomed N. Differential practice of treating ankle arthritis in a general and specialty orthopaedic society. American Orthopaedic Foot and Ankle Society: 20th Annual Summer Meeting. Seattle, July 29-31, 2004:Final Program 20:62.
3. Cornelis Doets H, van der Plaat LW, Klein JP. Medial malleolar osteotomy for the correction of varus deformity during total ankle arthroplasty: results in 15 ankles. Foot Ankle Int 2008;29(2):171–7.
4. Haskell A, Mann RA. Ankle arthroplasty with preoperative coronal plane deformity: short-term results. Clin Orthop Relat Res 2004;424:98–103.
5. Kopp FJ, Patel MM, Deland JT, et al. Total ankle arthroplasty with the Agility prosthesis: clinical and radiographic evaluation. Foot Ankle Int 2006;27:97–103.
6. Knecht SI, Estin M, Callaghan JJ, et al. The Agility total ankle arthroplasty. Seven to sixteen-year follow-up. J Bone Joint Surg Am 2004;86:1161–71.
7. Spirt AA, Assal M, Hansen ST Jr. Complications and failure after total ankle arthroplasty. J Bone Joint Surg Am 2004;86:1172–8.
8. Valderrabano V, Hintermann B, Dick W. Scandinavian total ankle replacement: a 3.7-year average followup of 65 patients. Clin Orthop Relat Res 2004;424:47–56.
9. Wood PL, Deakin S. Total ankle replacement. The results in 200 ankles. J Bone Joint Surg Br 2003;85:334–41.
10. Culpan P, Le Strat V, Piriou P, et al. Arthrodesis after failed total ankle replacement. J Bone Joint Surg Br 2007;89:1178–83.
11. Kitaoka HB. Salvage of nonunion following ankle arthrodesis for failed total ankle arthroplasty. Clin Orthop Relat Res 1991;268:37–43.
12. Thomason K, Eyres KS. A technique of fusion for failed total replacement of the ankle: tibio-allograft-calcaneal fusion with a locked retrograde intramedullary nail. J Bone Joint Surg Br 2008;90:885–8.
13. Myerson MS, Won HY. Primary and revision total ankle replacement using custom-designed prostheses. Foot Ankle Clin 2008;13:521–38.
14. Kharwadkar N, Harris NJ. Revision of STAR total ankle replacement to hybrid AES-STAR total ankle replacement—a report of two cases. Foot Ankle Surg 2009;15:101–5.
15. Assal M, Greisberg J, Hansen ST Jr. Revision total ankle arthroplasty: conversion of New Jersey Low Contact Stress to Agility: surgical technique and case report. Foot Ankle Int 2004;25:922–5.
16. DiDomenico LA, Williams K. Revisional total ankle arthroplasty because of a large tibial bone cyst. J Foot Ankle Surg 2008;47:453–6.
17. Pyevich MT, Saltzman CL, Callaghan JJ, et al. Total ankle arthroplasty: a unique design. Two to twelve-year follow-up. J Bone Joint Surg Am 1998;80:1410–20.
18. Myerson MS, Mroczek K. Perioperative complications of total ankle arthroplasty. Foot Ankle Int 2003;24:17–21.
19. Saltzman CL, Amendola A, Anderson R, et al. Surgeon training and complications in total ankle arthroplasty. Foot Ankle Int 2003;24:514–8.
20. Schuberth JM, Patel S, Zarutsky E. Perioperative complications of the Agility total ankle replacement in 50 initial, consecutive cases. J Foot Ankle Surg 2006;45: 139–46.

21. Hintermann B, Valderrabano V, Dereymaeker G, et al. The HINTEGRA ankle: rationale and short-term results of 122 consecutive ankles. Clin Orthop Relat Res 2004;424:57–68.
22. Saltzman CL, Mann RA, Ahrens JE, et al. Prospective controlled trial of STAR total ankle replacement versus ankle fusion: initial results. Foot Ankle Int 2009;30: 579–96.
23. Hanson TW, Cracchiolo A 3rd. The use of a 95 degree blade plate and a posterior approach to achieve tibiotalocalcaneal arthrodesis. Foot Ankle Int 2002;23: 704–10.
24. Buechel FF Sr, Buechel FF Jr, Pappas MJ. Ten-year evaluation of cementless Buechel-Pappas meniscal bearing total ankle replacement. Foot Ankle Int 2003;24:462–72.
25. Criswell BJ, Douglas K, Naik R, et al. High revision and reoperation rates using the Agility(TM) total ankle system. Clin Orthop Relat Res 2012;470:1980–6.
26. Labek G, Klaus H, Schlichtherle R, et al. Revision rates after total ankle arthroplasty in sample-based clinical studies and national registries. Foot Ankle Int 2011;32:740–5.

Polyarticular Sepsis Originating from a Prior Total Ankle Replacement

Sara L. Borkosky, DPM[a], Michael Mankovecky, DPM[b],
Mark Prissel, DPM[b], Thomas S. Roukis, DPM, PhD[c],*

KEYWORDS

- Osteomyelitis • Infection • Implant • Joint replacement • Revision

KEY POINTS

- Advances in technology for total ankle arthroplasty implants have increased the popularity of this procedure as an alternative to ankle arthrodesis.
- Deep periprosthetic infection remains a potential complication even with appropriate aseptic surgical technique.
- Infection involving the prosthetic components are limb threatening and can lead to polyarticular joint sepsis, which can quickly become life threatening.
- With adherence to basic principles of medical stabilization and surgical intervention in a staged manner with excision of all infected, necrotic tissue, a functional limb can be restored.
- Close follow-up within a multidisciplinary approach is required to monitor for signs of recurrent infection or loss of stability.

INTRODUCTION

With the development of current-generation implants, total ankle arthroplasty has regained popularity as an alternative to arthrodesis for end-stage ankle arthritis.[1] However, despite advances in technology and surgical technique, deep periprosthetic infection remains a possible complication. This problem is limb threatening, and requires timely intervention and often removal of components to gain control.[2,3]

Financial disclosure: None reported.
Conflict of interest: None reported.
[a] PGY-III, Gundersen Lutheran Medical Foundation, Mail Stop C03-006A, 1900 South Avenue, La Crosse, WI 54601, USA; [b] PGY-II, Gundersen Lutheran Medical Foundation, Mail Stop C03-006A, 1900 South Avenue, La Crosse, WI 54601, USA; [c] Department of Orthopaedics, Podiatry, and Sports Medicine, Gundersen Lutheran Healthcare System, 2nd Floor, Founders Building, Mail Stop FB2-009, 1900 South Avenue, La Crosse, WI 54601, USA
* Corresponding author.
E-mail address: tsroukis@gundluth.org

Clin Podiatr Med Surg 30 (2013) 97–100
http://dx.doi.org/10.1016/j.cpm.2012.08.007
0891-8422/13/$ – see front matter © 2013 Elsevier Inc. All rights reserved.

Although rare, as demonstrated through this case study, an infected total ankle arthro-plasty can evolve to polyarticular sepsis and if treatment is delayed, multisystem organ failure can ensue. This article presents a case of an 80-year-old man initially seen with left lower extremity cellulitis that progressed to polyarticular sepsis, deep peripros-thetic infection, and multisystem organ failure.

SURGICAL TECHNIQUE

Following medical stabilization, the patient underwent serial irrigation and debride-ment procedures for deep periprosthetic infection of his left total ankle arthroplasty and left total knee arthroplasty, in addition to septic bilateral wrists. All sites healed uneventfully, except the left total ankle arthroplasty, which underwent additional failed attempts at wound closure. The patient was referred to the senior author for further care and presented with incisional dehiscence anteriorly, desiccated anterior tibial tendon, and cardinal signs of recalcitrant deep periprosthetic infection (**Fig. 1**A). The patient underwent a protocol-driven approach consisting of wide resection of all infected, necrotic tissue, including the anterior tibial, extensor hallucis longus, and extensor digitorum longus tendons, with removal of lateral plate and screw fixa-tion, and the ultrahigh-molecular-weight polyethylene insert (**Fig. 1**B).[2–4] In addition to broad-spectrum parenteral antibiotics, polymethylmethacrylate antibiotic loaded beads were implanted and negative pressure-wound therapy was undertaken (**Fig. 1**C).[5] Repeat irrigation, debridement, bead exchange, and replacement of the negative pressure-wound therapy dressing was performed 48 hours later, which revealed a clean, healthy wound bed with no residual infection (**Fig. 2**A). Subse-quently, complex layered wound closure with split-thickness skin graft from the ipsi-lateral thigh was performed with bone marrow aspirate concentrate from the proximal tibia (**Fig. 2**B, C).[6–9]

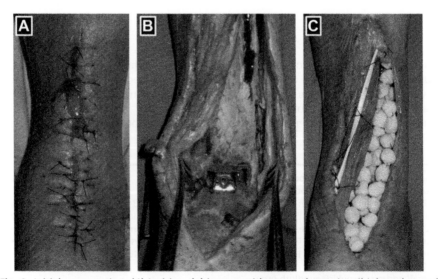

Fig. 1. Initial presentation. (*A*) Incision dehiscence with exposed anterior tibial tendon and purulent drainage. (*B*) Wide debridement of all nonviable tissue with polyethylene compo-nent removed. (*C*) Implantation of antibiotic loaded polymethylmethacrylate beads with use of Hunter rod.

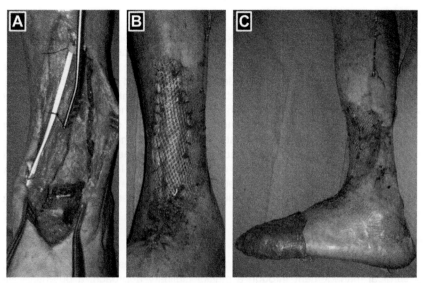

Fig. 2. Repeat irrigation and debridement at 48 hours. (*A*) Clean, healthy wound bed with no residual infection; split-thickness skin graft wound coverage harvested from ipsilateral thigh. (*B*) Anteroposterior view. (*C*) Lateral view.

CLINICAL OUTCOME

The patient was monitored closely throughout the postoperative course during which time uneventful healing of the incision with incorporation of the split-thickness skin graft occurred. At 2-year follow-up there are no signs of recurrent infection (**Fig. 3**). In addition, his ankle remains stable and functional, despite the ultrahigh-molecular-weight polyethylene insert not having been replaced at the time of final closure.

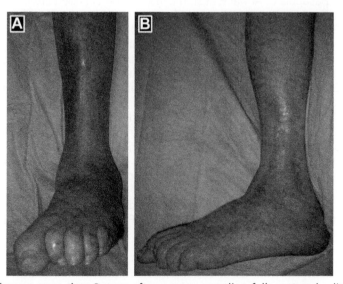

Fig. 3. Follow-up more than 2 years after surgery, revealing fully matured split-thickness skin graft with no evidence of residual infection. (*A*) Anteroposterior view. (*B*) Lateral view.

COMPLICATIONS AND CONCERNS

A multidisciplinary team approach is required to closely monitor a patient with deep periprosthetic joint sepsis, especially in the setting of retained implant hardware. The patient has been followed every 2 to 3 months by the senior author to assess the ankle for any recurrent skin breakdown that could lead to ulceration and deep-seeded infection. In addition, the infectious disease specialists involved in his care have initiated lifelong suppression with oral antibiotics. Ongoing peripheral edema owing to restricted range of motion and the nature of the original infection require continuous treatment. Compression stockings and refraining from prolonged leg dependency when the patient is not actively ambulating help to limit the extent of peripheral edema. With the assistance of the primary care team, oral diuretics have been prescribed and adjusted as needed. Finally, close monitoring is needed to assess for loss of stability to the ankle joint and for assessment of any need for bracing.

SUMMARY

This case demonstrates that by adhering to basic principles of medical stabilization and surgical management through a multidisciplinary approach, a potentially life-threatening infection involving polyarticular sepsis, deep periprosthetic infection, and multisystem organ failure can be successfully managed. In addition, a protocol-driven approach to deep periprosthetic infection allowed achievement of a retained, stable, functional, and noninfected total ankle replacement in this elderly patient.

REFERENCES

1. Guyer AJ, Richardson EG. Current concept review: total ankle arthroplasty. Foot Ankle Int 2008;29:256–64.
2. Sia IG, Berbari EF, Karchmer AW. Prosthetic joint infections. Infect Dis Clin North Am 2005;19:885–914.
3. Kotnis R, Pasapula C, Anwar F, et al. The management of failed ankle replacement. J Bone Joint Surg Br 2006;88:1039–47.
4. Levin LS. Debridement. Tech Orthop 1995;10:104–8.
5. Schade VL, Roukis TS. The role of polymethylmethacrylate antibiotic-loaded cement in addition to debridement for the treatment of soft tissue and osseous infections of the foot and ankle. J Foot Ankle Surg 2010;49:56–62.
6. Levin LS. The reconstructive ladder: an orthoplastic approach. Orthop Clin North Am 1993;24:393–409.
7. Roukis TS. Skin grafting techniques for open diabetic foot wounds. In: Zgonis T. Surgical reconstruction of the diabetic foot and ankle. Philadelphia: Lippincott Williams & Wilkins; 2009. p. 129–39.
8. Schweinberger MH, Roukis TS. Percutaneous autologous bone-marrow harvest from the calcaneus and proximal tibia: surgical technique. J Foot Ankle Surg 2007;46:411–4.
9. Schade VL, Roukis TS. Percutaneous bone marrow aspirate and bone graft harvesting techniques in the lower extremity. Clin Podiatr Med Surg 2008;25:733–42.

Current Concepts and Techniques in Foot and Ankle Surgery

Salvage of a Failed DePuy Alvine Total Ankle Prosthesis with Agility LP Custom Stemmed Tibia and Talar Components

Thomas S. Roukis, DPM, PhD

KEYWORDS

• Osteomyelitis • Infection • Implant • Joint replacement • Revision

KEY POINTS

• The Agility total ankle replacement system has been in clinical use for nearly 20 years.
• Revision of a failed Agility total ankle replacement is a challenge, with little published guidance available.
• Exchange of the Agility total ankle replacement components to a larger size, to the newer LP design, to custom stemmed components, or conversion to another ankle replacement system are considerations.
• Custom-designed Agility LP total ankle arthroplasty is unfortunately no longer available owing to US Food and Drug Administration regulation.

INTRODUCTION

The Agility total ankle replacement system (DePuy Orthopedics, Warsaw, IN), with the use of polymethylmethacrylate cement fixation, was the only implant approved by the Food and Drug Administration in the United States from 1998 to 2007.[1–8] Although not definitive, the incidence of revision, defined as component replacement, arthrodesis, or amputation[9] after primary implantation of the Agility total ankle replacement system over this time period, has recently been determined to be 9.7% (224 revisions out of 2312 primary implants) at a weighted mean follow-up of 22.8 months.[8] However, after the first phase of development between 1983 and 1993 during which the implant was exclusively used and modified by the inventor Frank G. Alvine, a select group of orthopedic foot and ankle surgeons around the United States had access to the DePuy

Financial Disclosure: None reported.
Conflict of Interest: None reported.
Department of Orthopaedics, Podiatry and Sports Medicine, Gundersen Lutheran Healthcare System, second Floor Founders Building, Mail Stop FB2-009, 1900 South Avenue, La Crosse, WI 54601, USA
E-mail address: tsroukis@gundluth.org

Clin Podiatr Med Surg 30 (2013) 101–109
http://dx.doi.org/10.1016/j.cpm.2012.08.008   podiatric.theclinics.com
0891-8422/13/$ – see front matter © 2013 Elsevier Inc. All rights reserved.

Alvine Total Ankle Prosthesis between 1993 and 1995, and provided continued feedback.[1-6,8] Although the exact fate of these DePuy Alvine implants is not known,[1-8,10-20] a mean 9-year follow-up of 132 implants between 1984 and 1994 revealed that 14 (11%) required revision in the form of component exchange or arthrodesis.[5] Revision of any phase of the Agility system to a custom-designed prosthesis has only infrequently been published as a treatment option.[21-27]

This article presents a case of revision of a phase 2 version of the DePuy Alvine Total Ankle Prosthesis to a custom-designed stemmed tibial and talar component Agility LP Total Ankle Replacement System.[28] The patient sustained a left-sided pronation-abduction ankle fracture dislocation following a fall from a height and underwent open reduction with internal fixation in 1994. He developed distal-lateral tibial osteonecrosis and advanced degenerative joint disease that was debilitating. Following removal of the retained deep internal fixation, he underwent primary implantation of a size-3 DePuy Alvine Total Ankle Prosthesis at age 56 years. The tibial component subsequently developed severe subsidence with anterior angulation, and the talar component developed subsidence with varus angulation (**Fig. 1**). Clinical examination revealed severely restricted sagittal plane range of motion with an osseous end to both dorsiflexion and plantarflexion motion. Significant lateral ankle instability was also appreciated, emanating from the ankle and subtalar joint. He was initially treated with functional brace therapy and lateral insole wedging that failed to provide any meaningful relief. He was counseled on operative intervention consisting of either tibio-talo-calcaneal arthrodesis or revision total ankle replacement with conversion to the INBONE or INBONE II Total Ankle Replacement System (Wright Medical Technologies, Inc, Memphis, TN) with lateral ankle stabilization, or the Agility LP custom-design stemmed total ankle replacement system (DePuy Orthopedics, Warsaw, IN) with lateral ankle stabilization. The patient refused an arthrodesis as a first-line revision treatment option. The choice between the revision total ankle replacement systems was based on the need to resect a significant portion of the distal tibia to expose

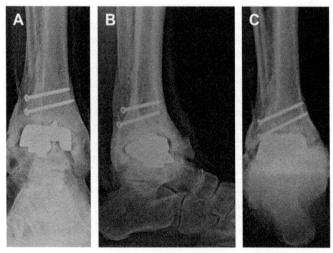

Fig. 1. Weight-bearing anterior-posterior (A), lateral (B), and hindfoot alignment (C) radiographs demonstrating extensive syndesmosis arthrodesis, aseptic osteolysis, and gross loosening of the tibial and talar components, with severe subsidence of the tibial component into the distal tibial metaphysis and severe varus deformity of the hindfoot originating from the ankle.

healthy bone and to extend the talar component fixation into the calcaneus for additional support following resection of a significant portion of the talar body. The INBONE or INBONE II total ankle replacement system would have required the use of revision ultrahigh-molecular-weight polyethylene (UHMPE) inserts and, therefore, limited future revision options. In addition, no long stem secured to the talar component is commercially available for the INBONE or INBONE II systems, and the use of metal reinforced polymethylmethacrylate cement augmentation of the talus[29,30] is still in the experimental stage. For these reasons it was determined that creation of an Agility LP custom-design stemmed tibial and talar component total ankle replacement with lateral ankle stabilization was most appropriate.

In brief, the design process for the Agility LP custom-design stemmed tibial and talar components involved obtaining a specific computed tomography imaging sequence of the entire hindfoot and ankle to allow for accurate determination of necessary height augmentation, sizing, and angulation of the stemmed components, and planned UHMPE thickness based on the level of planned osseous resection following removal of the failed ankle replacement (**Fig. 2**). In addition to the custom-designed Agility LP stemmed tibial and talar component total ankle replacement system including porous coating of the stems and horizontal surfaces, a custom stemless trial talar component with tunnel for guide-wire placement to align the talar component stem, and a trial custom stemmed talar component are included in the custom services with the trial components, coming with reusable insertion handles (**Fig. 3**).

SURGICAL TECHNIQUE

Under general anesthesia with a popliteal block, the previous anterior ankle incision, overlying the extensor hallucis longus tendon and the junction between this tendon

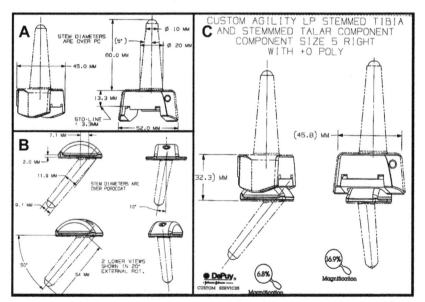

Fig. 2. Custom tibial and talar component template demonstrating the lateral and anterior-posterior views of the stemmed tibial component with base augmentation to match the tibial bone defect (*A*), lateral and anterior-posterior views of the stemmed talar component with LP design (*B*), and articulated stemmed tibial and talar LP components with +0-mm UHMPE insert (*C*). (*Courtesy of* T.S. Roukis, DPM, PhD, La Crosse, WI.)

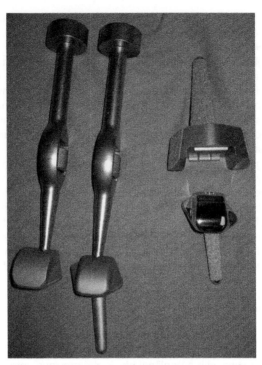

Fig. 3. From left to right, custom stemless trial talar component with tunnel for guide-wire placement secured onto insertion handle, custom stemmed trial talar component secured onto insertion handle, and final custom stemmed tibial (*top*) and talar (*bottom*) implants with porous coating on both stems, tibial external side walls, superior tibial component, and inferior talar component.

laterally and the tibialis anterior tendon maintained within its sheath medially, was developed and carried down to the underlying tibial and talus. Resection of scar tissue and inflamed synovium allowed visualization of the failed DePuy Alvine Total Ankle Prosthesis (**Fig. 4**A). Following removal of the failed ankle replacement system, the tibia and talus were prepared for acceptance of the custom stemmed tibial and talar components, being certain to adhere to the planned preoperative extent and alignment for resection to correct the varus deformity and anterior subsidence of the tibia, including the anterior tibial cortical window for stem placement (**Fig. 4**B). Following osseous preparation of the tibia, including cutting through the imbedded syndesmosis fusion screws, to accept the custom stemmed tibial component (**Fig. 5**A), the posterior, medial, and lateral aspects of the tibia were coated with antibiotic impregnated polymethylmethacrylate cement, and before curing the custom stemmed tibial component was imbedded, making certain that frontal plane angulation, transverse plan rotation, and axial height were maintained according to the preoperative template (**Fig. 5**B). A thin layer of antibiotic-impregnated polymethylmethacrylate cement was applied to the undersurface of the previously resected anterior tibial window, and this was press-fitted onto the tibial stem until the cement cured. The custom stemless trial talar component with tunnel for guide-wire placement to align the talar component stem was used under image intensification to align the drill for the talar stem, followed by sequential reaming until the trial custom stemmed talar component was able to be

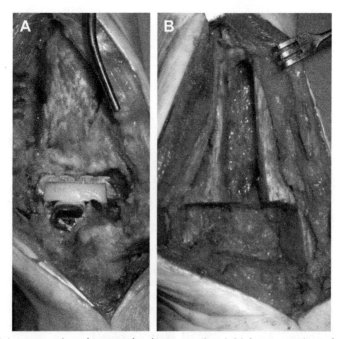

Fig. 4. (A) Intraoperative photographs demonstrating initial presentation of the Depuy Alvine Total Ankle Prosthesis following resection of the anterior tibial bone engulfing the implant. (B) Status following planar resection of the talar dome to correct varus malalignment deformity and resection of the distal tibia to accept the custom stemmed tibial component. It was necessary to cut through the screws used to perform the syndesmosis arthrodesis, as they had been completely overgrown with bone and could not otherwise be removed.

press fit. The custom stemmed talar component was then inserted with a thin layer of antibiotic-impregnated polymethylmethacrylate cement. The trial UHMPE insert was placed and deemed to consist of the 1+ design to achieve appropriate stability. As expected preoperatively, the lateral ankle complex was incompetent, and it was deemed necessary to perform a modified Evans whole peroneus brevis tendon transfer to achieve stability to inversion stress (**Fig. 5C**). This maneuver was performed following insertion of the final +1 UHMPE insert and involved a small incision at the musculotendinous junction at the lateral lower leg to transect the peroneus brevis tendon. The peroneus brevis tendon insertion to the fifth metatarsal base was maintained and the tendon was passed deep against the calcaneus, lateral talus, and anterior-lateral ankle where it was secured underneath the medial screw and plate used to further stabilize the anterior tibial cortical window. Following the modified Evans whole peroneus brevis transfer, the ankle maintained neutral alignment and achieved lateral-ankle stability against maximum inversion stress (**Fig. 5D**).

Throughout the procedure the surgical site was irrigated with copious amounts of sterile saline impregnated with antibiotics using a power lavage system. The surgical site was closed in layers over a suction drain and initially stabilized with a plaster splint. On the third postoperative day the drain was removed and a short-leg fiberglass cast was applied, with the foot held in neutral alignment relative to the lower leg. Serial dressing and cast changes occurred over the next 8 weeks followed by use of

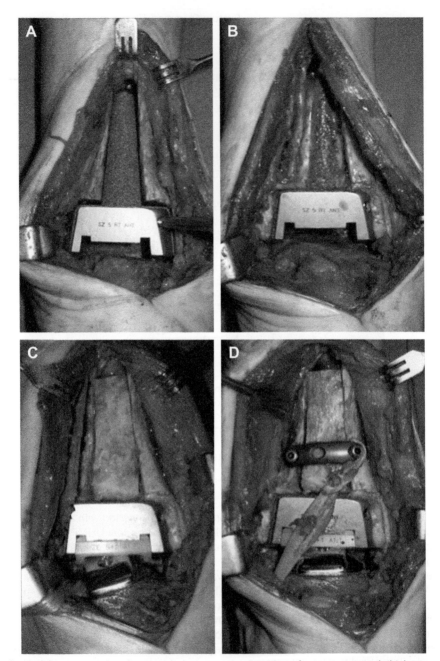

Fig. 5. (*A*) Intraoperative photograph demonstrating insertion of custom stemmed tibial component with handle used to maintain frontal and transverse plane alignment. (*B*) The custom stemmed tibial component is shown following antibiotic impregnated polymethylmethacrylate cement stabilization in the desired position. (*C*) The previously resected anterior tibial cortical window has been replaced, the custom stemmed talar component has been inserted following antibiotic impregnated polymethylmethacrylate cement stabilization in the desired position, and a +1 UHMPE insert has been placed. Note that despite the corrective resection of the talar dome and vertical placement of the custom stemmed talar component in the calcaneus, the ankle demonstrates persistent lateral ankle instability that requires stabilization. (*D*) Final alignment following transfer of the peroneus brevis tendon from the fifth metatarsal base to the medial distal tibia underneath the 3-hole plate-and-screw construct used to stabilize the anterior tibial cortical window. Note that the ankle is well aligned and is no longer laterally unstable to maximum inversion stress.

a removable pneumatic controlled ankle motion boot for an additional 8 weeks. The patient remained non–weight bearing for 12 weeks and gradually increased the distance ambulating on full weight for an additional 4 weeks. Gradual return to supportive shoe gear followed.

CLINICAL OUTCOME

Except for some expected rebound peripheral edema once immobilization began, no untoward complications occurred and the patient progressed to return of full ambulation and nonimpact exercise. At follow-up more than 1 year after final recovery the patient has a well-aligned, stable, and pain-free custom stemmed revision ankle replacement, with acceptable sagittal pane ankle range of motion to allow for unimpeded gait (**Fig. 6**).

COMPLICATIONS AND CONCERNS

The patient continues to undergo routine oral antibiotic prophylaxis for dental procedures. In addition, he avoids ambulation on uneven ground and ballistic activities including extensive ambulation.

Revision lateral ankle stabilization can be performed with the use of an allogenic tendon graft or split peroneus longus tendon transfer, to perform a Chrisman-Snook type repair. The longevity of the Agility LP custom stemmed tibial and talar total ankle replacement remains uncertain. Conversion to an INBONE or INBONE II total ankle replacement system will be a challenge, given the current cemented nature of the custom stemmed tibial component and extensive bone loss to both the tibia and talus. Tibio-talo-calcaneal arthrodesis, even with massive amounts of autogenous

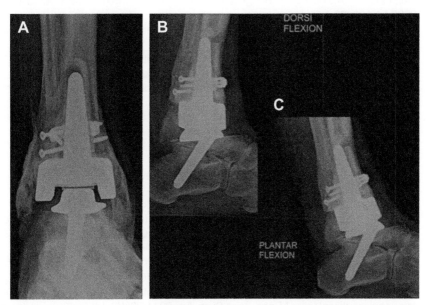

Fig. 6. Weight-bearing anterior-posterior view (A), and lateral stress dorsiflexion (B) and stress plantarflexion (C) views demonstrating maintained alignment of the custom stemmed tibial and talar components, with good sagittal-plane range of motion of the ankle and no tendency toward varus malalignment.

corticocancellous bone graft, will be a challenge for these same reasons. Unfortunately, any custom-designed Agility total ankle replacement is not currently available for clinical use owing to US Food and Drug Administration regulation, and the availability of this hardware in the future remains uncertain.

SUMMARY

This article presents a case whereby a second-phase design DePuy Alvine Total Ankle Prosthesis underwent revision to an Agility LP design custom-stemmed tibial and talar component total ankle replacement system. The rationale for this procedure, the process of developing the custom components, the operative sequence of events, and recovery course are presented in detail. Causes for concern regarding subsequent revision, should this be required, are raised.

REFERENCES

1. Alvine FG. Total ankle arthroplasty: new concepts and approach. Contemp Orthop 1991;22(4):397–403.
2. Alvine F. Design and development of the agility ankle. Foot Ankle Spec 2009;2(1): 45–50.
3. Alvine FG. The Agility ankle replacement: the good and the bad. Foot Ankle Clin 2002;7:737–53.
4. Pyevich MT, Saltzman CL, Callaghan JJ, et al. Total ankle arthroplasty: a unique design. Two to twelve-year follow-up. J Bone Joint Surg Am 1998;80(10):1410–20.
5. Knecht SI, Estin M, Callaghan JJ, et al. The Agility total ankle arthroplasty: seven to sixteen-year follow-up. J Bone Joint Surg Am 2004;86(6):1161–71.
6. Salzman CL, Alvine FG. The Agility total ankle replacement. Instr Course Lect 2002;51:129–33.
7. Rippstein PF. Clinical experiences with three different designs of ankle prosthesis. Foot Ankle Clin 2002;7:817–31.
8. Roukis TS. Incidence of revision after primary implantation of the Agility total ankle replacement system: a systematic review. J Foot Ankle Surg 2012;51:198–204.
9. Henricson A, Carlsson Å, Rydholm U. What is revision of total ankle replacement. Foot Ankle Surg 2011;17:99–102.
10. Guyer AJ, Richardson G. Current concepts review: total ankle arthroplasty. Foot Ankle Int 2008;29(2):256–64.
11. DeOrio JK, Easleu ME. Total ankle arthroplasty. Instr Course Lect 2008;57: 383–413.
12. Gougoulias NE, Khanna A, Maffulli N. History and evolution in total ankle arthroplasty. Br Med Bull 2009;89:111–51.
13. Smith TW, Stephens M. Ankle arthroplasty. Foot Ankle Surg 2010;16:53.
14. Gougoulias NE, Khanna A, Maffulli N. How successful are current ankle replacements? A systematic review of the literature. Clin Orthop Relat Res 2010;468: 199–208.
15. van den Heuvel A, Van Bouwel S, Dereymaeker G. Total ankle replacement: design evolution and results. Acta Orthop Belg 2010;76:150–61.
16. Easley ME, Adams SB, Hembree WC, et al. Current concepts review: results of total ankle arthroplasty. J Bone Joint Surg Am 2011;93(15):1455–68.
17. Haddad SL, Coetzee JC, Estok R, et al. Intermediate and long-term outcomes of total ankle arthroplasty and ankle arthrodesis. J Bone Joint Surg Am 2007;89(9): 1899–905.

18. SooHoo NF, Zingmond DS, Ko CY. Comparison of reoperation rates following ankle arthrodesis and total ankle arthroplasty. J Bone Joint Surg Am 2007; 89(10):2143–9.
19. Labek G, Thaler M, Janda W, et al. Revision rates after total joint replacement: cumulative results from worldwide joint register datasets. J Bone Joint Surg Br 2011;93(3):293–7.
20. Labek G, Klaus H, Schlichtherle R, et al. Revision rates after total ankle arthroplasty in sample-based clinical studies and national registries. Foot Ankle Int 2011;32(8):740–5.
21. Myerson MS, Won HY. Primary and revision total ankle replacement using custom-designed prosthesis. Foot Ankle Clin 2008;13:521–38.
22. Haddad SL. Revision agility total ankle arthroplasty. Chapter 76. In: Easley Mark E, Wiesel Sam W, editors. Operative techniques in foot and ankle surgery. Philadelphia: Lippincott Williams & Wilkins; 2011. p. 622–42.
23. Myerson MS. Revision total ankle replacement. Chapter 25. In: Myserson Mark S, editor. Reconstructive foot and ankle surgery: management of complications. 2nd edition. Philadelphia: Elsevier Saunders; 2010. p. 295–316.
24. Vienne P, Nothdurft P. OSG-totalendoprosthese agility: indikationen, operationstechnik und ergebnisse. Fuss Sprungg 2004;2:17–28 [in German].
25. Gould JS. Revision total ankle arthroplasty. Am J Orthop (Belle Mead NJ) 2005; 34(8):361.
26. Alvine FG, Conti SF. Die agility-sprunggelenkprothese: mittel- und langfristige erfahrungen. Orthopäde 2006;35:521–6 [in German].
27. Steck JK, Anderson JB. Total ankle arthroplasty: indications and contraindications. Clin Podiatr Med Surg 2009;26:303–24.
28. Cerrato R, Myerson MS. Total ankle replacement: the agility LP prosthesis. Foot Ankle Clin 2008;13:485–94.
29. DeOrio JK. Total ankle replacement with subtalar arthrodesis: management of combined ankle and subtalar arthritis. Tech Foot Ankle Surg 2010;9:182–9.
30. Schuberth JM, Christensen JC, Rialson JA. Metal-reinforced cement augmentation for complex talar subsidence in failed total ankle arthroplasty. J Foot Ankle Surg 2011;50:766–72.

Diabetic Calcaneal Fractures

Bryan A. Sagray, DPM[a], John J. Stapleton, DPM[b,c],
Thomas Zgonis, DPM[a,*]

KEYWORDS

- Diabetes • Calcaneal fractures • Neuropathy • Charcot neuroarthropathy • Arthrosis

KEY POINTS

- Acute traumatic fractures in the diabetic patient can also lead to the development of Charcot neuroarthropathy, of which the exact mechanism is controversial.
- A poor soft tissue envelope associated with an open fracture or fracture blisters, whether serous or hemorrhagic, needs to be treated in an efficient and expedited manner.
- Primary subtalar joint arthrodesis for severely comminuted diabetic calcaneal fractures may be obtained by the use of a circular external fixation or by using limited incisions and percutaneous internal fixation techniques.

INTRODUCTION

The incidence of treating calcaneal fractures among diabetic patients continues to increase, as does the percentage of the population diagnosed with diabetes mellitus. Therefore, systemic manifestations of the disease along with the fracture pattern have to be considered when formulating a treatment plan. Many factors have been associated with predisposition to foot fractures in the diabetic patient, particularly decreased bone density. Causes may include long-term prednisone for immunosuppression, renal osteodystrophy, or postrenal transplant.[1] Significant loss of bone mass in diabetic patients can be appreciated as early as 5 years after diagnosis.[2] This situation is further compounded by decreased cortical bone integrity and dysfunction of bone metabolism.[3,4] Acute, traumatic fractures in the diabetic patient can also lead to further episodes of Charcot neuroarthropathy, of which the exact mechanism is controversial.

Most calcaneal fractures are caused by a fall from a height. Falls or jumps from ladders, scaffolds, and roofs have been the cause of most of these injuries. In addition,

[a] Division of Podiatric Medicine and Surgery, Department of Orthopaedic Surgery, University of Texas Health Science Center at San Antonio, 7703 Floyd Curl Drive MSC 7776, San Antonio, TX 78229, USA; [b] Foot and Ankle Surgery, Lehigh Valley Hospital, Cedar Crest Campus, 1250 South Cedar Crest Boulevard, Suite 110, Allentown, PA 18103, USA; [c] Penn State College of Medicine, 500 University Drive, Hershey, PA 17033, USA
* Corresponding author.
E-mail address: zgonis@uthscsa.edu

Clin Podiatr Med Surg 30 (2013) 111–118
http://dx.doi.org/10.1016/j.cpm.2012.09.001   **podiatric.theclinics.com**

calcaneal fractures are infrequently seen in motor vehicle accidents. Calcaneal fractures are typically the result of high-energy trauma with a direct axial load or sudden eccentric contracture of the Achilles tendon. However, in the diabetic patient with decreased bone density or neuropathy, calcaneal fractures can occur from reported low-energy falls and with various mechanisms of injury. Calcaneal fractures can be easily overlooked in the diabetic patient, because the typical presentation of severe pain and inability to bear weight may be altered secondary to peripheral neuropathy, if present. The clinical findings of edema and ecchymosis with a history of trauma to the heel in a diabetic patient should raise a high index of suspicion for a calcaneal fracture.

Regardless of the cause, fracture management in diabetic patients must consider the soft tissue envelope, the vascularity of the extremity, and the need for prolonged fracture stabilization.[5]

The incidence for secondary arthrodesis among diabetic patients is not known, but the percentage might be less because pain scores are lower in patients with diabetic peripheral neuropathy. For this reason, overall fracture management in the diabetic population should be mainly focused on avoiding major complications and providing fracture stabilization. A recent meta-analysis confirms that operative treatment of calcaneal fractures better restores anatomic structure and leads to better functional outcomes; however, this comes with high likelihood of complications.[6] These complications include wound dehiscence, infection, joint arthrosis, painful hardware, nerve injury, and risk for limb loss. In addition, the diabetic patient with dense peripheral neuropathy presents an even further challenge to these operative complications, and further surgical techniques may need to be implemented for the treatment of diabetic calcaneal fractures.

CLINICAL FACTORS ASSOCIATED WITH DIABETES MELLITUS

Diabetes mellitus has a significant effect on soft tissue and bone healing, increasing the chance of nonunion and wound complications in patients with fractures or undergoing attempted arthrodesis.[7,8] Many different factors combine to negatively influence tissue healing, several of which are commonly found in the diabetic patient: immunosuppression, chronic anemia, renal insufficiency, coronary artery disease, peripheral neuropathy, and peripheral vascular disease.[9] A specific treatment plan is patient-dependent and may include but is not limited to closed reduction with cast immobilization, closed reduction with percutaneous skeletal stabilization, open reduction with internal fixation, external fixation, or any combination of techniques.

Numerous studies have been published reporting an increased time to complete osseous union in diabetic patients undergoing fracture repair. One such study[8] found that diabetic patients with displaced fractures or fractures undergoing open reduction and internal fixation required 187% and 186% more time to unite, respectively. Another study[10] proved that radiological and functional outcomes were drastically altered in the diabetic patient, with malunion occurring 18.7 times more often. A strong correlation has also been found between diabetics and soft tissue complications. One study of closed fractures treated nonoperatively in diabetics compared with nondiabetics, found infection rates of 32% and 8.8%, respectively.[11] Complication and infection rates can reach as high as 91.6% when peripheral vascular disease and neuropathy accompany the diabetic patient.[12] The detrimental effects of uncontrolled hyperglycemia are well established for other diabetic comorbidities, but have more recently been extrapolated to fracture and soft tissue healing. When comparing diabetic patients with 1 or more of the following comorbidities (smoking, need for renal

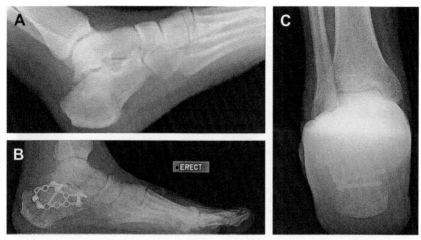

Fig. 1. Preoperative lateral (*A*) view of an intra-articular joint depressed calcaneal fracture in a well-controlled diabetic patient without any related complications. Final postoperative lateral (*B*) and calcaneal axial (*C*) views, showing anatomic alignment after an open reduction and internal fixation was performed through an extensile lateral approach.

dialysis, peripheral vascular disease, and previous foot ulcerations), a well-controlled hemoglobin A1c was most predictive of successful healing.[13]

SURGICAL MANAGEMENT OF DIABETIC CALCANEAL FRACTURES

The initial evaluation begins with a thorough evaluation for multiple traumatic injuries that can occur from high-energy trauma. Life-threatening conditions such as head injury, chest, or abdominal and pelvic injuries need to take priority in treatment. Common contiguous fractures associated with calcaneal fractures involve the spine, contralateral extremity, and the wrist. The diabetic patient without any comorbidities and with optimal glycemic control is typically treated in the same manner as a patient without diabetes mellitus. However, the diabetic patient with poorly controlled hyperglycemia and diabetic-related complications requires further assessment, which may alter treatment.

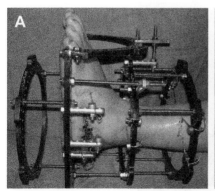
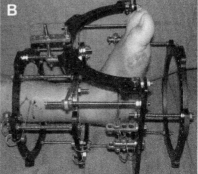

Fig. 2. Postoperative clinical lateral (*A*) and medial (*B*) views of a common circular external fixation device for the management of calcaneal fracture repair or primary arthrodesis of the talocalcaneal joint with limited incision placement or percutaneous fixation.

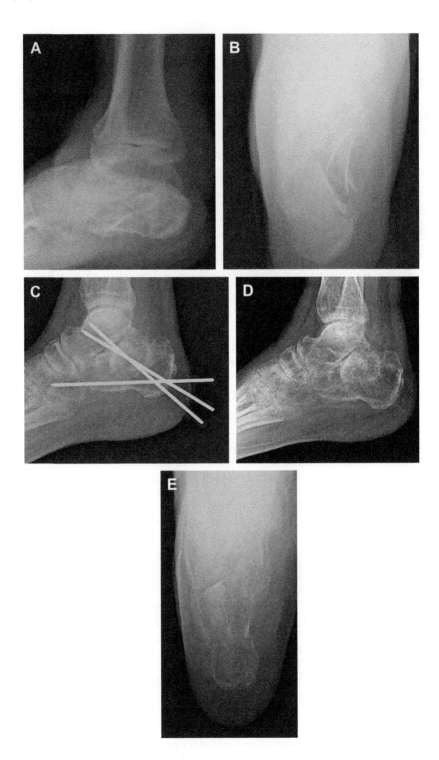

Evaluation of the lower extremity focuses primarily on the neurovascular supply to the foot, degree of soft tissue injury, presence of open wounds, infection, compartment syndrome, and obvious deformity/dislocation. A lower extremity vascular assessment begins with determining the presence or absence of a palpable dorsalis pedis and posterior tibial artery. Doppler studies or angiography may be obtained if needed. The presence of peripheral arterial disease is more prevalent among diabetic patients and smokers. Arterial injury, although rare, can be associated with high-energy trauma and especially with open calcaneal fractures or calcaneal fractures combined with a dislocation or significantly displaced medial calcaneal wall. Significant arterial occlusive disease based on these parameters requires vascular surgery consultation for possible revascularization options and to guide further treatment regarding fracture management.

A detailed neurologic lower extremity examination can be performed in responsive patients. The tibial nerve can be injured and initial evaluation determines if plantar sensation is present. Patients with diabetes and peripheral neuropathy may have loss of plantar sensation related to diabetic peripheral neuropathy, and evaluating the contralateral extremity can provide insight into whether peripheral neuropathy is present. In addition, the lack of pain in the diabetic patient with a calcaneal fracture should also be a clinical finding that suggests the presence of peripheral neuropathy. Compartment syndrome as a result of increased pressure with the subcalcaneal and foot compartments may be present and can also alter sensation. A high index of suspicion is necessary, especially in the diabetic patient with peripheral neuropathy, because the presence of severe pain out of proportion is typically not present. Often, severe edema with tenting of the skin and positive intracompartmental pressure measurements are the only clinical parameters available to make the diagnosis in diabetic patients with peripheral neuropathy.

Assessing the extent of soft tissue injury is paramount in determining a time frame and surgical approach to achieve fracture reduction. An open reduction and internal fixation through an extensile lateral approach requires an optimal soft tissue envelope, decreased edema, healing of fracture blisters, positive pinch test, and presence of skin wrinkles (**Fig. 1**). Surgical approaches that involve limited incisions and percutaneous techniques typically are performed in an acute manner to achieve fracture reduction through these techniques, despite a less than optimal soft tissue envelope (**Fig. 2**). The notion in these clinical case scenarios is that limited incisions should be less likely to develop wound complications compared with an extensile approach but need to be performed acutely to facilitate fracture reduction. Delaying surgical intervention can lead to the inability to achieve adequate fracture reduction through closed reduction or limited incisional techniques.

Open diabetic calcaneal fractures pose significant risk for deep infection and limb loss. Initial management requires thorough irrigation and surgical debridement of the

---

Fig. 3. Preoperative lateral (A) and calcaneal axial (B) views, showing a severely comminuted and dislocated open calcaneal fracture in a diabetic patient with a poor soft tissue envelope and neurovascular compromise. Postoperative lateral (C) view, showing the calcaneal fracture reduction that was achieved through the open medial wound and stabilized with percutaneous Steinmann pins. Delayed primary closure of the wound was performed within 48 hours after the initial irrigation and surgical debridement. The Steinmann pins were used as the definitive method of fixation to minimize the risk of wound healing complications and were removed at 10 weeks postoperatively. Final lateral (D) and calcaneal axial (E) views, showing interval healing and satisfactory alignment.

wound, if feasible. At the time of initial surgical debridement of the open fracture, major fracture fragments should be manipulated and repositioned through the open wound to prevent further compromise to the soft tissue envelope. At times, the use of Steinmann pins placed percutaneously or application of an external fixator is advantageous to maintain this reduction (**Fig. 3**). The goal of this initial stage is not to achieve anatomic reduction but to improve the overall alignment of the calcaneus to facilitate healing of the surrounding soft tissues, which is particularly important in the diabetic population. In certain clinical case scenarios, definitive reduction in the diabetic patient population may consist of this limited surgical approach to achieve healing of both the soft tissue and bone and minimize the risk of major complications. Immediate intravenous antibiotics are initiated and continued according to standard protocols for open fracture management. The presence of infection with open diabetic calcaneal fractures requires adequate surgical debridement, removal of loose and unstable hardware if present, and obtaining intraoperative cultures to guide parenteral antibiosis. Delayed reconstructive procedures can be performed only after eradication of infection.

Plain radiographic evaluation combined with computed tomography (CT) is necessary to evaluate the fracture pattern. CT scans are most useful in evaluating calcaneal fractures. CT images can be obtained in 2-mm intervals in the axial, sagittal, and 30° semicoronal planes. CT images with three-dimensional reconstructive views are beneficial in pulverized fracture patterns. Understanding the pathoanatomy is required to formulate a surgical approach to achieve surgical reduction. Based on the fracture pattern and associated soft tissue injury, reduction can be achieved either indirectly with a traction table and external fixation or directly through an open reduction and internal fixation with the traditional lateral extensile approach.[14] Indirect reduction techniques can provide minimal incision approaches, because wound healing complications tend to be increased in the diabetic population.[15] After reduction of the fracture fragments, a minimal sinus tarsi incision is placed laterally to allow for direct exposure of the talocalcaneal joint to perform a primary arthrodesis or fracture repair. For primary arthrodesis, the remaining articular cartilage is denuded and bone graft may be added to promote osseous consolidation. Primary subtalar joint arthrodesis for the severely comminuted diabetic calcaneal fractures may be obtained by the use of a circular external fixation or by combining percutaneous internal fixation. Additional large-diameter transarticular Steinmann pins may also be used for fracture stabilization.

The use of circular external fixation provides a multitude of benefits, including reduction and stability of the fracture, promoting compression at the arthrodesis site if performed, augmenting limited internal fixation if inserted, and simultaneously off-loading and protecting the soft tissue envelope. The circular external fixator may also be placed as a simple off-loading type device when internal fixation is used as a primary method of fixation.[16]

In general, patients are kept nonweight bearing to the operative extremity until consolidation is noted on follow-up radiographs. If an external fixator was applied, it is then removed once the soft tissue or bone healing is achieved, depending on the reason the external fixator was used, and the patients are then allowed progressive weight bearing as tolerated in a removable walking boot or cast, with additional instructions from physical therapy. At that point, supportive shoe gear or bracing may be necessary and patients are followed at designated postoperative intervals.

DISCUSSION

The outcomes of surgically treated diabetic calcaneal fractures are poorly understood, with most of the literature being extrapolated from diabetic ankle fractures. However, there does seem to be a clear consensus that early diagnosis and treatment are crucial to preventing significant bony deformity.[1]

External fixation has been extensively studied for limb lengthening, angular and post-traumatic deformity correction, and trauma surgery. Many of these same benefits can be applied to the diabetic patient with a calcaneal fracture, regardless of its being acute or neuropathic in nature. The application of a Delta-frame construct was shown to provide a viable alternative to the traditional open reduction and internal fixation method, by using the theory of ligamentotaxis without the need of large surgical dissection.[17] Several recent articles have discussed open reduction with internal fixation or spanning external fixation as a first staged approach to reducing long-term complications associated with comminuted intra-articular calcaneal fractures. Radnay and colleagues[18] advocated operative treatment initially because it provided better functional outcomes and lower complication rates when a talocalcaneal arthrodesis was performed at a later date for posttraumatic arthrosis. Popelka and Simko[19] had similar results when they treated first with external fixation and then with an arthrodesis.

As stated earlier, many factors predispose the diabetic patient to an increased risk/rate of complications after operative intervention of calcaneal fractures. These factors may include and are not limited to osteopenic bone, previous renal or pancreas transplantation, immune dysfunction, and tissue hypoxia resulting from small/large blood vessel disease, increased viscosity of hyperglycemic blood, and impaired oxygen delivery by glycosylated hemoglobin.[20]

SUMMARY

The ideal treatment recommendations for calcaneal fractures in the diabetic patient remain controversial and continue to evolve. Further clinical studies and research in the management of diabetic calcaneal fractures can provide guidelines and outcomes in this patient population.

REFERENCES

1. Hedlund LJ, Maki DD, Griffiths HJ. Calcaneal fractures in diabetic patients. J Diabetes Complications 1998;12:81–7.
2. Levin LS, Nunley JA. The management of soft tissue problems associated with calcaneal fractures. Clin Orthop 1993;290:151–6.
3. Piepkorn B, Kann P, Frost T, et al. Bone mineral density and bone metabolism in diabetes mellitus. Horm Metab Res 1997;29:584–91.
4. Leidig-Bruckner G, Ziegler R. Diabetes mellitus: a risk for osteoporosis? Exp Clin Endocrinol Diabetes 2001;109:493–515.
5. Schon LC, Easley ME, Weinfeld SB. Charcot neuroarthropathy of the foot and ankle. Clin Orthop Relat Res 1998;349:116–31.
6. Jiang N, Lin Q, Diao X, et al. Surgical versus nonsurgical treatment of displaced intra-articular calcaneal fracture: a meta-analysis of current evidence base. Int Orthop 2012;6:1615–22.
7. Cozen L. Does diabetes delay fracture healing? Clin Orthop 1972;82:134–40.
8. Loder RT. The influence of diabetes mellitus on the healing of closed fractures. Clin Orthop 1988;232:210–6.
9. Kagel EM, Einhorn TA. Alterations of fracture healing in the diabetic condition. Iowa Orthop J 1996;16:147–52.
10. Chahal J, Stephen DJ, Bulmer B, et al. Factors associated with outcomes after subtalar arthrodesis. J Orthop Trauma 2006;20:555–61.

11. Flynn JM, Rodriguez-del Rio F, Piza PA. Closed ankle fractures in the diabetic patient. Foot Ankle Int 2000;21:311–9.
12. Costigan W, Thordarson DB, Debnath UK. Operative management of ankle fractures in patients with diabetes mellitus. Foot Ankle Int 2007;28:32–7.
13. Younger AS, Awwad MA, Kalla TP, et al. Risk factors for failure of transmetatarsal amputation in diabetic patients: a cohort study. Foot Ankle Int 2009;30:1177–82.
14. Zgonis T, Roukis TS, Polyzois VD. The use of Ilizarov technique and other types of external fixation for the treatment of intra-articular calcaneal fractures. Clin Podiatr Med Surg 2006;23:343–53.
15. Mehta SK, Breitbart EA, Berberian WS, et al. Bone and wound healing in the diabetic patient. Foot Ankle Clin 2010;15:411–37.
16. Facaros Z, Ramanujam CL, Zgonis T. Primary subtalar joint arthrodesis with internal and external fixation for the repair of a diabetic comminuted calcaneal fracture. Clin Podiatr Med Surg 2011;28:203–9.
17. Kissel CG, Husain ZS, Cottom JM, et al. Early clinical and radiographic outcomes after treatment of displaced intra-articular calcaneal fractures using delta-frame external fixator construct. J Foot Ankle Surg 2011;50:135–40.
18. Radnay CS, Clare MP, Sanders RW. Subtalar fusion after displaced intra-articular calcaneal fractures: does initial operative treatment matter? Surgical technique. J Bone Joint Surg Am 2010;92:32–43.
19. Popelka V, Simko P. Surgical treatment of intra-articular calcaneal fractures. Acta Chir Orthop Traumatol Cech 2011;78:106–13.
20. Prisk VR, Wukich DK. Ankle fractures in diabetics. Foot Ankle Clin North Am 2006; 11:849–63.

Index

Note: Page numbers of article titles are in **boldface** type.

Clin Podiatr Med Surg 30 (2013) 119–122
http://dx.doi.org/10.1016/S0891-8422(12)00156-5
0891-8422/13/$ – see front matter © 2013 Elsevier Inc. All rights reserved.

podiatric.theclinics.com

Moving?

Make sure your subscription moves with you!

To notify us of your new address, find your **Clinics Account Number** (located on your mailing label above your name), and contact customer service at:

Email: journalscustomerservice-usa@elsevier.com

800-654-2452 (subscribers in the U.S. & Canada)
314-447-8871 (subscribers outside of the U.S. & Canada)

Fax number: 314-447-8029

Elsevier Health Sciences Division
Subscription Customer Service
3251 Riverport Lane
Maryland Heights, MO 63043

*To ensure uninterrupted delivery of your subscription, please notify us at least 4 weeks in advance of move.

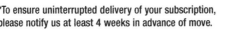

Printed and bound by CPI Group (UK) Ltd, Croydon, CR0 4YY

03/10/2024

01040440-0015